Yoga for Beginners

by

Swami Gnaneswarananda

Edited and Compiled by

MALLIKA CLARE GUPTA

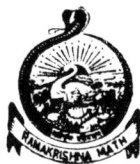

SRI RAMAKRISHNA MATH

16, Ramakrishna Math Road,
Madras-600 004.

Published by
Adhyaksha
Sri Ramakrishna Math
Mylapore, Chennai-4

First Edition, March 1976
Twelfth Print, October 2015
2M3C

ISBN 81-7823-314-2

**Total number of copies
printed till now: 24,900**

Printed in India at
Sri Ramakrishna Math Printing Press
Mylapore, Chennai-4

PUBLISHER'S NOTE

We have great pleasure in presenting to our readers the Indian edition of **Yoga for Beginners** by Swami Gnaneswarananda.

Yoga is a term to conjure with. It has come to mean many things to many men. Swami Gnaneswarananda, who founded the Vivekananda Vedanta Society in Chicago, has taken enormous pains to explain the essence of traditional Yoga in a concise, lucid and lovely language, shorn of all technicalities. His up-to-date phraseology laced with humour can be understood and enjoyed by all enquiring minds. The Swami has based his expositions on the great dictum of Swami Vivekananda: "Each soul is potentially divine. The goal is to manifest this divinity within, by controlling nature, external and internal. Do this either by work, or worship, or psychic control, or philosophy—by one, or more, or all of these—and be free."

In clear and persuasive language, Swami Gnaneswarananda has sketched the four great paths to God-realization:

Karma Yoga —Perfection through work.
Bhakti Yoga —Perfection through Love.
Raja   Yoga —Perfection through meditation.
Jnana Yoga —Perfection through knowledge.

We are sure that the readers will find the book eminently helpful in their spiritual practice.

Originally, these lectures appeared serially in the pages of the *Vedanta Kesari* published by this Math. Later they were brought out in book form by the Vivekananda Vedanta Society of Chicago. We are grateful to the Society for permission to bring out this Indian Edition.

Sri Ramakrishna Math, Madras   **PUBLISHER**
March, 1976.

PREFACE

As THE title indicates, this book is primarily intended for beginners in spiritual life. However, those who are well along the road to spiritual achievement will also find much encouragement and inspiration in it. *Yoga for Beginners* is a compilation of the spoken words of Swami Gnaneswarananda as they were taken down, mostly stenographically, by three of his students, Virginia Knapik, Genevieve Spoonholtz, and myself over a period of some years.

In a compilation of this sort there are bound to be some repetitions and reiterations. But I think that these enhance rather than detract from the book's value. The subjects discussed require a great deal of attention on the part of the reader. Repetition of an idea is, therefore, very helpful. A good teacher will naturally repeat and explain in different ways the subject of discussion, in order to better reach the mind of the student.

Swami Gnaneswarananda's yoga classes were held Tuesday evenings on the premises of the Vedanta Society of Chicago, then located at 120 East Delaware Place. The Swami would give his talks seated at a small table, with the students sitting around him. This made the classes very informal. The Swami spoke extemporaneously, introducing many lively stories and anecdotes to bring out his points and to enliven discussion. He was thus able to put before his students the highest religious and philosophical teachings of the Hindu religion in a language and idiom they could really understand. To paraphrase Swami Vivekananda, he could take a person from wherever he stood and lift him up.

One did not have to have high academic qualifications in order to understand Swami Gnaneswarananda. The Swami's manner of teaching, in fact, was so simple that it was only after some reflection that one could fully appreciate its depth. One of the Swami's strongest convictions was that knowledge does not come from outside us. It is an unfoldment from within. The duty of the teacher in any field of knowledge, he would say, was to stimulate the mind of the student and help him to remove the *inner* obstructions to the perfect unfoldment or realization of that knowledge.

Swami Gnaneswarananda was a person of great charm, with a magnetic personality. He had a boyish nature, with a smile for everyone and an enthusiasm for spiritual endeavour that was contagious. He was equally at home discussing the intricacies of philosophy with the elders or telling stories of the saints and sages to small children, fascinating them with his tales. Two qualities seemed most prominent in his nature: a spiritual love that enveloped all beings in the universe; and a dynamic approach to, and understanding of, the problems that aspirants in spiritual life have to cope with.

"The clearest and most open thing in the world," the Swami once said, "is the means to attain divine life; but because of our passions and weaknesses we have covered that up with all sorts of 'secret knowledge' and lots of other nonsense. The 'open sesame' to spiritual life is the secret of being and becoming, of having the strength and courage to carry a thing into actual practice, no matter how simple and devoid of high-sounding and befooling names it may be. This is the 'open secret' knowing which we can wake up from this long and painful world-dream. There is no short-cut to that.

"Truth is always simple. It is only falsehood that is intricate and complicated. Spirituality is simplicity. I find that many people are interested in yoga, particularly Saja Yoga. But most of them have a very odd conception of what it really is. Many think that it is something magical, like Aladdin's lamp, something that can bring them, without the least trouble, all the things they wish to enjoy. They learn a couple of postures and a few peculiar ways of breathing and right away they become Aladdins of the twentieth century, even without a lamp! To others it appeals as the builder of perfect health and enduring beauty. Do whatever you like, live any way you please, only learn some yogic tricks and then you are free from indigestion, headache and overweight. And lo! Look into your mirror and see what magic charm your features radiate.

"These are all complexes. Only when everything about a person has become simple can the truth reveal itself in its simplest and healthiest form. It is weakness of the brain that gathers mystery around Yoga. Yoga is not for the weak. What we want is mysticism without the 'mist.' I consider it my business to bring all types of 'magic' into the penetrating light of knowledge, so that whatever is fake in them will vanish and whatever is real and true will gain the precision of scientific knowledge. I therefore earnestly request you to cast from your minds all notions of mystery and magic regarding Yoga Spiritual unfoldment does not mean the achievement of any supernatural or magical powers. Far from it!''

Every effort has been made to weave these notes, sometimes taken down at random, into a whole that is both comprehensive and representative of the Swami's Yoga classes. It is hoped that this little book will reach the hearts of sincere aspirants in spiritual life and that in it they will find much to ponder over and much to enjoy. The search for spiritual perfection should be accompanied by ioy, even laughter, and not by a morose, "sackcloth and ashes" attitude!

The compiler wishes to acknowledge with gratitude the permission given by the *Vedanta Kesari,* Madras, India, to reproduce these notes in their present form. They first appeared in that magazine in serial form from November, 1967, through May, 1971.

Mallika Clare Gupta

CONTENTS

		PAGE
Preface		v
Publisher's Note		viii
Introduction		1
I.	JNANA YOGA: *the Path of Knowledge*	13
II.	RAJA YOGA: *the Path of Psychological Control*	93
III.	BHAKTI YOGA: *the Path of Love*	126
IV.	KARMA YOGA: *the Path of Selfless Work*	156
V.	A SUMMING UP	186
	Glossary	201
	Index	209

INTRODUCTION

SWAMI VIVEKANANDA summed up the whole of religion in three statements:

1. Each soul is potentially divine.
2. The goal is to manifest this divinity within, by controlling nature—external and internal.
3. Do this either by work, or worship, or psychic control, or philosophy, by one, or more, or all of these—and be free.

"This is the whole of religion," added Swami Vivekananda. "Doctrines, or dogmas, or rituals, or books, or temples, or forms, are but secondary details."

Let us consider these statements as three propositions.

PROPOSITION 1: *Each soul is potentially divine.*

What is meant by the term, "divinity"? Most people have a very vague notion about this. Divinity is an existence which is infinite, immortal, imperishable; absolute, all-knowing, all-powerful, and ever-blissful. The word, divinity, therefore, implies the state of (1) absolute existence, (2) unlimited power, (3) infinite knowledge, and (4) eternal bliss. Any conception of divinity, of God, or of an ultimate state or being, must include these attributes. Such a divinity, God, ultimate state or being must be perfect, and in order to be perfect it must be of the nature we have just described. Divine perfection is uncaused, unlimited, and un-conditioned by time, space, or causation.

In relation to man what do I mean by divinity? I mean that highest ideal of perfection which we all want to attain in the course of our lives. I mean the unfoldment of that state of consciousness in which we will have no defect, misery, suffering, or limitation of any kind. Spontaneously, knowingly or unknowingly, we all respond to an urge for that. What are we all working for? What is our highest goal in life? In short, we are all working for the attainment of the ideal state of perfection, for the attainment of limitless existence, absolute knowledge, and infinite happiness.

We want to *live*. And we want to live in such a way that there will not be any suffering, disease, death, or an imperfection of any kind disturbing our existence.

We want to *know*. We spontaneously feel that we have a right to attain a state where there will not be anything in this universe unknown to us. We are all looking for that state of realization. Our discoveries, inventions, and all the advancement of intellectual thought and scientific progress have been possible owing to that inner urge in man.

We spontaneously feel that we have a right to be *happy*. Of course, the philosophy underlying the ideal and the method for the attainment of that state of bliss might be different with different individuals. But, so far as the fundamental urge is concerned, it is one and the same for everyone.

The motive force behind every living being is a similar fundamental urge for the unfoldment of the state of perfect existence, knowledge, and bliss. We do not have to be taught about this state of divinity, for it is not without; *it is always within*.

Can you find any living being who does not like to live? Can you find a man who has honestly become reconciled to disease and death? Where is the person who is satisfied with the state of imperfection? Can we become reconciled to ignorance? Why this insatiable yearning for more and more knowledge? There is no human being who does not feel a deep sense of protest against the state of ignorance. Tell a human being that he has no right to know, and see how insulted he feels. Why such sensitiveness?

What about happiness? There are people who have been suffering all their lives. But were they reconciled to their state of misery? Were they not always looking for that "silver lining" to the dark cloud of their suffering, either in this life or in a life hereafter? This shows that in man's inner nature there is a firm conviction that he has the *right* to be happy.

Man's instinctive protest against imperfection of any kind—against death, ignorance, suffering, and so on—presupposes that he is born with the unshakable conviction that infinite perfection is his birthright. That man is divine is shown by his response to this conviction and his resentment towards the contrary, spontaneously and intuitively.

The subjective ideal of perfection, of divinity, has been concretized and objectified in the form of a personal   conception of divinity, or God. If you speak to people about God being possessed of these divine attributes—absolute existence, knowledge, and bliss—they will agree. But when you speak of *their* inner divinity they often seem shocked. Analyze your conception of God and you will find that it is nothing but the concretized picture of the fulfillment of absolute existence, knowledge, and bliss. God does not become old or sick; he does not die. He knows everything; there is no limitation to his knowledge. God has the capacity for the enjoyment of infinite bliss. Nothing can make him sad or depressed. These are the three basic subjective ideals that have been concretized, objectified, and developed into the conception of an objective deity.

Why is it that most of you are ready to agree that these ideals describe God, or an ultimate being or state, but are not so ready to agree that these may be ascribed to the nature of man also? Why do you hesitate to believe that man is potentially divine? First of all let me ask you that if divinity is infinite, which it must be, will it not pervade everything? Will there be any place where it is not? Could there be anything else besides divinity? No. Because if there were, the infinite would not be infinite. Infinite implies the existence of one only. The existence of anything else would limit it and it would lose its infinite nature.

There are three sources of knowledge, or means by which truth may be verified: authority, inference, and direct perception. Let us consider these.

AUTHORITY. This means reliable authority, from persons who have realized the truth themselves, or from scriptures or other records of those who have realized the truth. Ninety percent of all our knowledge is gained from this source. For instance, we say we know and we accept as true many scientific facts. But have we, ourselves, experimented and proved them? We have not. We accepted the authority of those who have experimented and reached certain conclusions which they have proved to themselves to be true. We may, in the same way, accept the findings of those in authority in spiritual matters if they have experimented and gained direct perception of the truth. This should satisfy the most scientific "modern."

INFERENCE. There are several items to be considered under this heading:

a) *Change presupposes the existence of the Unchangeable.* In order for change to be recognized it must be observed by someone who is, relatively, less changing. The subject, *S*, sees the object, *A*, changing into A-1, *A*-2, *A*-3, *A*-4, and so on (the figures representing time). If the subject, *S*, were not relatively less changing than the object, no change in the object could be discerned. However, the subject, *S*, may be observed by another subject which watches *S* as a changing object. If we were to continue this analysis *ad infinitum*, directing our attention first to the object and then to the subject, we would find the same process operating. Therefore, we must admit that there is, ultimately, one which is constant, in order for change to be recognized at all. That which is changeless is eternal, infinite. Where is there any other to work change upon it? The changeless is perfect and, therefore, divine. You cannot logically impute change to divinity.

(*b*) *The distinctness of the subject-object consciousness.* Consider this in regard to your self, and your body and mind. Divinity is within you, but you do not know it because you have taken your self for something which it is not. What do you mean by your "self"? It is the body, the mind, the intellect, the emotions, or other faculties? No. You have the clear consciousness of these being *used by you*. You are conscious that you have a mind. Being conscious of anything presupposes that we are something other than the thing we are conscious of. "My body, my mind," you say. You know that you are not the body, yet in the next instant if the body becomes ill you think you are the body. Such is your inconsistency! You say, "I think, I discriminate," and so on. You know you are not the mind or the functions of the mind. Who is the subject of all these changing states of your body and mind, including the state of deep and dreamless sleep?

Are you your coat? No, you possess your coat. Who is the possessor of the body, mind, and all the faculties? Where is the possessor? Consider the subject-object consciousness, the relationship of possessor and possessed, in regard to the body, the mind, and the real Self. That which is the possessor cannot be the same as the possessed.

(*c*) *The nature of compounds.* A compound exists for something which does not form a part of the compound. First, consider it within the microscosm. The human entity is made up of three "bodies," according to Hindu philosophy. They are the gross, physical body; the mental "body", consisting of the ego-consciousness, the mind, and so on; and the causal "body", which is the most subtle of the three and which holds the seed of world-consciousness. This compound of the three bodies (called *sarira*, in Sanskrit, meaning "that which changes") exists for the benefit of the Self of man, which is beyond them. These three bodies are sometimes called sheaths, or coverings, of the soul.

It is possible to break all compounds into their component parts. This process, as regards material life, is what is known as disintegration or death. The existence of any compound which is subject to change presupposes an unchangeable, simple entity. Only that which is beyond causation, which cannot be acted upon, can be unchangeable. Therefore, it follows that only perfection or omnipotence can be strictly unchangeable, can be purely " simple".

The Divinity, being uncaused and immutable, is a "simple" entity. It cannot be compounded by anyone or anything, or for anyone's benefit. It is not made up of parts brought together as in a manufactured object. It is, in its very nature, the witness of all compounds, of all combinations, and combinations of combinations. Divine perfection is uncaused, is ever-all-itself and, therefore, it can never vanish, can never not be.

(*d*) *Evolution presupposes involution.* The seed is the tree involved; the tree, the seed evolved. If you sow the seed of a mango it will not be possible for you to grow an apple tree. You can only get an apple tree from an apple seed. The potentiality of the giant tree is within the little seed; the potentiality must be there for it to manifest. The child is the man involved; the man, the child evolved.

Take a mechanical illustration. The effect is the cause manifest; it is the cause in another form. You get the amount of power out of an engine from the amount of causes you put into it, causes in the form of water, coal, gas, fire, and so on. If the materials are not there you cannot get the motive force you expect from it. If the potentiality of perfection were not in man he could not talk, or even think, about perfection. If it were wholly absent from his nature it would be absolutely impossible for any-one to discuss, much less to manifest, perfection or divinity. We can only become what we potentially are.

If a single being ever overcame imperfection it must logically be inferred that that perfection was *within him*. If, in one single instance. perfection was expressed by a human being, that perfection was certainly contained in the cause, or the fundamental human nature. We believe that Christ, Krishna, Buddha (and I might mention dozen o.her persons) attained perfection. You, of course, do not think of Jesus the Christ as human, but we consider our prophets as such. Jesus of Nazareth became the Christ and manifested Christhood in his life. Buddha, for instance, was not born a Buddha; he was born with the inherent potentiality of Buddhahood. He manifested and exemplified in his life the manner in which Buddhahood could be realized, unfolded, and expressed. If the state of Buddhahood were not contained in him, it could never have been expressed by him. It was contained in the cause, the fundamental human nature.

Some put forward the argument that divinity is not within you, but that you may attain it after death in a place called heaven. In other words, divinity is not *innate*, but *acquired*. But what is our conception of perfection? That it is infinite, for who would be satisfied with finite perfection or happiness? Finite is that which may be taken away from you at any moment. It has its limitations. If divinity does not exist here and now, but will exist at a future time in another place, the conception of divinity is limited by time, space, and location. That is a self-contradiction. Hence, it is illogical. That which is infinite must be within you now, or it never will be. It must be everywhere or nowhere. Divinity can neither be attained by changing locations nor can it be bestowed upon one at some future time. *Now or never!*

The most conclusive proof of the existence of the Divinity within is that of experiment. When you make an experiment and demonstrate something for yourself, you get the best proof. When you go to a chemical laboratory and the teacher tells you that if you mix two parts of hydrogen with one part of oxygen and apply a spark you will get water, what is your proof of it? Experiment. The teacher speaks with authority because he has, himself, experimented and found the truth for himself. But what is your own proof? Direct, personal experience. Suppose you are taught the method of experiment to find out the divinity within and you take up that method and succeed in it. That will be the most conclusive proof. Direct perception is the third means of verifying truth.

DIRECT PERCEPTION. Direct perception, personal experience,

is the final proof. By following an authentic and systematic method of practice, the divinity can clearly be demonstrated. That, alone, is the most conclusive proof in this matter. Both inference and authority have to be resorted to in order to reach direct perception. All three of these basic sources of knowledge must unite to give the same verdict. When, by all three of these, a conclusion is reached, then it is true. That is, as far as human conception is concerned. These three means of verifying knowledge are called, in Hindu philosophy, *pramana*. (The life of Sri Ramakrishna showed all the different methods of arriving at the truth. His life itself was pramana).

PROPOSITION 2: *The goal is to manifest this divinity within, by controlling nature, external and internal.*

We are divine, but why do we not know it? Why do we feel so powerless to manifest it? Because there are certain obstacles in the way of its manifestation. These obstacles in the way of the manifestation of the Divinity within have to be removed. This is done by "controlling nature, external and internal." Life means the struggle of the soul to assert its own right. The purpose of life is to overcome the obstacles that prevent manifestation of the soul's real nature, which is divine perfection.

What are these obstacles? They are: (1) not-knowledge; (2) agitation of the mind-stuff ; (3) false self-consciousness; and (4) desire for possessions and attachment to them.

Not-knowledge means indiscrimination and illusion. In Sanskrit this is called *avidya*, that is, not-knowledge or ignorance as to the true nature, the divine nature, of man.

Ten men were once crossing a river. There was no ferry boat, so they had to swim across. The river was wide and deep, and it had a strong current. The man were not expert swimmers, so from the beginning they were fearful they might be carried away.

After much difficulty they reached the other side of the river. The leader gathered his group around him and began to count them in order to be sure they had all safely reached shore.

"One, two, three," he counted, "four, five, six, seven, eight, nine—" he stopped. "Alas," he cried, "the tenth is lost! The tenth is lost!"

The people sat down on the bank of the river and mourned the loss of their friend. After some time a stranger came upon the scene. He asked the people the reason for their sorrow. The leader of the group related the story of the lost man. The stranger glanced over the group and asked them to count again. The man did so and stopped as before, at nine, bursting into tears as he did so. "The tenth is lost! The tenth is lost!" he cried.

The stranger grabbed him and said: "My friend, *thou* art the *tenth!*"

We, like the man in the story, think that the state of our perfection is lost. We mourn the loss of it while all the time it is within us. Divinity is within us, yet all the time we are bewailing its loss. We have been carrying this perfection within us all the time, but because of our *misconception* of it we do not recognize it. What is actually needed is "disillusionment." We have to rouse ourselves out of the state of misconception. We have to wake up from our delusion. When the awakening comes, we realize our mistake. We find that through all our process of searching, we had been carrying within us the very thing we were searching for. We did not have the correct knowledge of the true nature of our Self. This is called avidya. Correct knowledge is *vidya*. (It is said that the musk deer carries in its navel the sweet-scented musk. It runs frantically here and there in the forest, trying to discover the source of that fascinating smell. Sometimes it even injures itself in doing so. It does not know that all the while it is carrying the musk within its own body.)

The *agitation of the mind-stuff* is called *chitta-vritti* in Sanskrit (*chitta*, consciousness, and *vritti*, ripples or waves). The agitation of the mind-stuff obstructs the manifestation of divinity. (Actually, nothing can obstruct divinity; it is our understanding of it, our vision, that is obstructed.)

Suppose you have a pool in your yard and you have made a beautiful marine garden. If the water is agitated or unclean how can you expect to see it? If there are ripples and little wavelets agitating the surface of the water you will not be able to see your marine garden. You want to look into the water and see the beautiful shells and attractive flora, the colorful fish swimming about. But until the water is calm, clean, and quiet you will see only the agitations. They will obstruct your view.

Your consciousness is the pool of water which contains the "marine garden" of divinity. If you would keep your consciousness transparent and unagitated you would realize the Divinity there. It is external stimuli, worldly thoughts and contacts, and the internal stimuli of desires, hopes, plans, memories, and so on, that keep our consciousness in a state of storm and tempest. How are we to attain that state of quietude? The method is simple enough to state: learn the art of keeping your mind calm and transparent. There is a special method by which this may be achieved.

False self-consciousness is another obstacle. In Sanskrit this self is called *ahamkara*, or the individualized ego-consciousness. So long as we associate ourselves with the little individualized ego, we cannot realize the Divinity. We have to give up this false self-consciousness.

Once a tigress, big with young, attacked a flock of sheep. In her strenuous attempt she was then and there delivered of a little cub. The mother died, however, and the tiger cub was raised among the flock of sheep. Although physically the little cub grew to be a full-grown tiger, yet in his consciousness he was nothing but a lamb. He behaved in every respect like a lamb. He bleated like a lamb, ate grass and was, like the lambs, afraid of other beasts, such as tigers. We may say that he became "self-hypnotized."

After a time another tiger from the forest fell upon that flock of sheep. He killed a little lamb and the rest were put to flight. To his utmost surprise, the tiger saw that among the fleeing sheep was a full-grown tiger, bleating in terror like the sheep. The tiger was very curious. He quickly overtook the self-hypnotized tiger, whom we shall call the tiger-lamb.

The tiger from the forest asked, "Why do you behave like this? Why do you act like a lamb?"

The tiger-lamb meekly replied, "Why, I *am* a lamb."

The big tiger said, "Nonsense! You are *not* a lamb. You are tiger, just as I am."

The tiger-lamb would not believe that. He was terribly frightened. Trembling in fear, he begged for his life. "Don't kill me," he implored.

The big tiger said, "I am not going to kill you, but I am going to kill that 'lamb-consciousness' in you. I want the 'tiger-consciousness' in you to be awakened. Come! I will show you that you are not a lamb, but a real tiger."

He drew the tiger-lamb near a pool of water and showed him his reflection. "See," he said, "Do you not look exactly like

G—2

me? Or, do you think you look like those lambs?"

The tiger-lamb looked and looked at his reflection in the pool of water and then at the big tiger from the forest. Consciousness began to dawn in him that he was not a lamb at all. He was a tiger! The tiger of the forest dragged him back to where he had left his prey. He told him, "Eat! Because you have been raised with those lambs and have been eating grass all this time, which is not the food of your race, you have forgotten your birthright. Come, I will initiate you into the food of your race. You must eat meat, and then the consciousness of the tiger will be fully awakened in you." The tiger-lamb hesitated, but the big tiger forced him to eat. Gradually, a transformation took place in the consciousness of the tiger-lamb.

The tiger of the forest told him to roar. He told him to imitate him. Oh, the thrill of joy the tiger-lamb now felt now in that mighty sound which once used to frighten him! There came forth from his throat the real, thundering roar of a tiger! The transformation was complete. As he dived into the forest, to live with his own kind, he roared in ecstasy.

We are all behaving like tiger-lambs. "Tigers" we are, divinities we are, but we have hypnotized ourselves into thinking we are weak mortal beings. We have to rid ourselves of this false self-consciousness. We must know we are just like the big "tiger," like God. We have to know that we are one with Him.

The *desire for possessions,* to keep and to add to one's possessions, is called *vasana.* We become attached to possessions, to the transitory things of life, and from this attachment a chain of causation is set in motion in which we become deeply enmeshed. It often becomes so complicated that we completely lose our way in the labyrinth of action. We cannot know our real nature until we rise above all action and attachment to action, and realize our self as being above these.

A man once took instruction from a wandering holy man. After a few days the holy man went away leaving his disciple to meditate in a hut on the outskirts of a small village.

The new monk would go out each day to beg his food. He would spend the rest of his time meditating, as instructed by his guru. One day, while he was away from the hut, a rat chewed up his loin cloth which he had washed and laid out in the sun to dry. Now, the monk had only one other loin cloth. The rat had left him with only the cloth he wore and a few shreds of the other one.

The next day when the monk went out to beg his food he mentioned his difficulty to some of the villagers. They were sympathetic and said, "Well, father, we can give you a new cloth today, but how can we give you a new cloth every day? Better get a cat. That will solve your rat problem."

The villagers gave him a cat and he took it to the hut with him. But he found that the cat made his life miserable, mewing day and night for milk. Meditation was impossible because of the cat.

The next day when he went to the village he asked for a little milk for the cat. The villagers said, "Well, father, we can give you some milk today, but it will be hard for us to supply you milk every day. Find a cow, then you will have plenty of milk for your cat." And they gave him a cow.

Then the monk found that he needed food for the cow. So someone gave him a plot of land where the cow could graze. This went on until he was surrounded by a small, prosperous farm. He was now very busy growing food for his cattle and for the farmhands and himself.

One day the holy man came back that way to see his disciple whom he had left meditating in the little hut. He wanted to see how far he had progressed with his practices. The holy man looked about him, surprised at seeing difference in the place. The hut was gone; there was a farm house in its place. The holy man saw some farm hands loitering nearby and asked them, "Can you tell me where that monk has gone who used to live here in a small hut?"

The disciple heard the voice of his guru and came running out of the farmhouse. The holy man stared at him. "What has happened to you, my son?"

The disciple told his story. The holy man shook his head sadly and said, "Ah! My son! And all for a piece of loin cloth!"

These, then, are the four basic obstacles to the manifestation, to the realization, of the Divine within. Now we come to the third proposition. How do we overcome the obstacles to the manifestation of the Divine within?

PROPOSITION 3. *Do this either by work, or worship, or psychic control, or philosophy, by one, or more, or all of these-and be free.*

Humanity may be classified under three broad groups: the

awakened, the ready-to-be-awakened, and those who are asleep. The awakened are those who are aware of their divine nature. They may not be *completely* aware of it, but they are awakened enough. Naturally, they are in the minority. Those who are "asleep" are quite happy with their lives as they are. They do not think beyond this little world of sense objects. They constitute the great majority of mankind. The ready-to-be-awakened are the aspirants in spiritual life.

Again, spiritual aspirants are classified under four psychological types, their general characteristics and sources of inspiration being: (1) the *discriminating, reasoning type.* A philosophical mind responds quickly to this process; (2) the *psychic type,* which responds more to mental stimuli than to sense stimuli; (3) the *devotional, loving type* which has a great capacity for feeling; and (4) the *active type.* Here the appeal is to man's energetic, outgoing propensities.

All these four types are equally important. The principle of the one cannot be applied to another. The systematic method of practice which each type follows for the achievement of the highest goal is called *yoga.* The word, yoga, is derived from the Sanskrit root, *yuj,* one meaning of which is to join, to unite, to yoke. Hence, the primary meaning of the word is the process by which an aspirant is joined, united, or yoked to his highest Ideal. It means the union of the imperfect self with the divine Self. Each of the yogas can lead an aspirant to the goal, independent of any of the other yogas. Technically, yoga is a special science which enables a seeker of truth to realize the goal. The discriminative type follows the path of *jnana yoga.* For the psychic type, *raja yoga* is prescribed. *Bhakti yoga* is suitable for the devotional type, and *karma yoga* is recommended for the active type. However, a general study and practice of the principles of all the yogas is recommended.

Know that all the yogas lead to the same goal. Do not feel too inclined towards only one of them and underestimate the others. Any yoga, followed to its logical conclusion, will lead you to the highest goal.

Hindu philosophy is unique in that it has different methods of experimentation. It may, therefore, be called scientific. One who cares to practise conscientiously can learn for himself and judge by his own results.

I

JNANA YOGA

The Path of Knowledge

1

Remove the veil of maya; know the truth regarding your self, the universe, and Brahman, and be free.

THAT is the method, the endeavour, and the goal according to jnana yoga. The veil of *maya* covers the truth of these three entities. It has to be removed. What is *Brahman*? It is One, Changeless, Infinite Existence. It is Divinity; it is God. The connotation of the word Brahman, however, conveys much more than that of the word God, as understood in dualistic philosophy. The word Brahman literally means "the mighty," that beyond which there can be nothing else. It is the eternal "unknowable" Subject. Yet it can be realized.

Hindu philosophy describes Brahman in negative language as "not this, not this" [*neti, neti*]. It is "not this" because the Infinite cannot be an object of the mind. Everything we know is cognized by the mind. Brahman can never be circumscribed by the mind or senses. Elimination (or confirming that Brahman is "not this, not this" with reference to objects of the mind and senses) is the process of realizing what Brahman is. The infinite, formless Brahman cannot be an object because it cannot be bound by the limitations of space, time, and causation. If you think of a form you have to put it in space. Then it would be bound by the limitation of space. As soon as you admit the limitation of space you also admit the limitations of time and causation. Those three are interdependent; they hang or fall together. So, Brahman the formless and infinite One is described as "not this, not this."

In more positive language, Brahman has been described as perfection: Existence-Knowledge-Bliss Absolute. The Hindu scriptures, reliable authorities, have declared it to be so.

Inference and reasoning have also proved it, and Brahman has
been realized as such by great seers and God-men throughout the
ages in the supersensuous state of consciousness, the highest *samadhi*.
And they have told us it is possible for us to verify this truth for
ourselves.

What is maya? Maya is the inscrutable power that obstructs
our understanding of the reality. We are deluded by nescience,
or ignorance of Brahman, through the influence of maya. The
word maya literally means a device, an artifice of Brahman or the
mode of its seeming manifestation. The word is also often
translated as simply "illusion." By the device of maya, Brahman,
the One, Changeless Existence, appears to us as the universe with
its manifold manifestations. It is something like an actor playing
a role on the stage. When he plays a part he appears to be that
character, but he is not. Maya is neither existence nor non-existence.
This is a statement of fact. Brahman is the Immutable Entity out
of which phenomena (by the subtle influence of maya) appear to
us to have been projected, although no change has every taken place
in the absolute nature of Brahman. This "appearance" of Brahman
as manifestation, as the many, is also known as maya.

We find a simple illustration of this in moving pictures. The
figures projected on the screen have no reality except that
produced by the light which is behind them. The modulations
of the vibrations of light produce the figures on the screen. Other
than that, they have no real existence. Their reality is light, nothing
but light. In a similar manner the reality of all manifested things
is Brahman. They may appear to be real but they depend entirely
upon the steady "light" of Brahman for their existence. Brahman
is the immutable "light principle" behind the universe. When
you understand this profound game of "light" you can enjoy the
cosmic "movie." But when you do not know its secret you feel
yourself at its mercy. You are then no better than a poor soccer
ball, one moment at the feet and the next on the heads of the players.

The real Self of man has all the attributes of divinity. It is
divine. This was discussed, to some extent, in the introduction
and it will be the subject of further discussion as we proceed. The
divinity of the Self can be proved by three means: reliable
authority reasoning and inference, and direct perception. The
student in jnana yoga is particularly concerned with these
processes.

The method of attaining perfection through jnana yoga is based on the philosophy of non-dualism. According to Hindu philosophy, there are three ways of viewing the truth: *dvaitavada* (dualism). *visishta-advaitavada* (qualified non-dualism), and *advaitavada* (non-dualism). These, in turn, are concerned with three questions: What is the nature of the ultimate reality? What is the nature of the universe? What is the nature of the human soul? The Sanskrit term for philosophy is *darsana sastra*, or that which governs and takes one through all the steps of spiritual practice, or *sadhana*. It establishs the truth and then shows the discipline or practice to attain it. The word darsana is from the root *dris*, "to see," meaning that which gives us the power to understand, so that we may see things as they *are*, and not as something else. Two processes are involved: right speculation and right thinking. Through these we reach a conclusion. But merely to reach a conclusion is not enough. We must *be and become* that which we have concluded from our philosophical speculation.

Darsana primarily concerns itself with two elements: *pramana* "that by which we establish the truth," and *prameya*, "that which we want to know." Earlier, we discussed pramana, which connotes three ways of verifying the truth: authority [*agama*], inference [*anumana*], and direct perception [*pratyaksha*].

Under prameya, there are four concerns: *srishti*, projection or genesis: *jagat*, the universe of phenomena (both the microcosm and macrocosm); *jiva*, the individualized self; and Brahman (or *Isvara*), the ultimate reality. We want to know what the Self is, that which perceives all this universe. We want to know what the universe is, or that which is perceived. And we want to know what the nature of the ultimate reality is, that which is the genesis of all.

The items under prameya are treated by all orthodox schools of Hindu philosophy. These fall under the three different philosophical approaches mentioned previously. It was Swami Vivekananda, by the way, who pointed out for the first time that these views (dualism, qualifid non-dualism, and non-dualism, or monism) are complementary to one another. Although apparently opposed, they are, in actuality, not so.

The philosophy of monism [*advaitavada*] comprises two schools of thought: the *ajatavada*, or the non-creation theory, and the *vivartavada*, or illusion theory. The philosophy of monism which is, in particular, known as *Vedanta,* was expounded in the Upanishads, scriptures which are considered to be the "cream" of Vedic knowledge. Monism was firmly re-established by the great philosopher and saint, Sankaracharya, in the eighth century; but the revival of advaita Vedanta actually began with the very erudite scholar, Gaudapada Acharya, the grand-guru of Sankara. Gaudapada established the ajatavada, the non-creation theory. He expressed it something like this: "Creation is nothing but a nightmare. Wake up! That is all that is necessary." But, nobody would listen to him; no one could understand him. He had only one disciple, Govindapada, who understood him. Gaudapada lived to be several hundred years old. He defied death. He would not go, he said, until his philosophy was accepted. But Yama, the king of death, got tired waiting for him. Gaudapada was told that his teachings would have to be made teachable soon!

One night Gaudapada had a vision in which he saw that a little boy of eight would come to him and would, in time, make his philosophy acceptable. He asked how he would recognize the boy. He was told that the boy would show a miraculous power of yoga, and he would write a wonderful commentary on his philosophy; he would also be the youngest *sannyasin* [monk] he ever saw. But he would not be his disciple; he would be Govindapada's. He was also told that after this little boy came he could safely depart this life in peace!

Meanwhile, in Malabar, in Southern India, a little prodigy of eight, Sankara, had indeed become a sannyasin and set out in search of the great acharya, Gaudapada. When he arrived at the *asrama* of Gaudapada, he found the sage in deep meditation. Nearby, the Narmada river was in flood and Sankara thought that it would drown Gaudapada before he could even pay his respects to him. So he commanded the river to stop. It did not and he said, "What! You disobey me? I will show you!" And, according to the story, he imprisoned the Narmada in his little water bowl.

The fish in the river were now in great distress and they made so much noise floundering around in the mud that it awakened Gaudapada from his meditation. Looking around, he saw Sankara standing there, his face glowing, scornfully looking at the Narmada in his little bowl! He knew that this was the little boy of his vision. Gaudapada asked Sankara to release the river as the fish were in great trouble. Then he gave him his work, the *karika* [commentary] on the *Mandukya Upanishad,* and asked him to read it. They retired for the night.

The next morning Sankara appeared with the commentary he had written on the teachings of Gaudapada. The old teacher was amazed to find how clearly his teachings had been set forth by this little boy of eight. Gaudapada told Sankara that he was destined to be the disciple of Govindapada, and happily went into the state of *mahasamadhi* from which there is no return.

The *ajatavada* of Gaudapada holds that there has never been any creation. Therefore no question of God, soul, or the universe should ever arise; all dualistic conceptions are but creations of dream. Brahman alone exists. The way to realize It is not by discussing the question, not by asking the "why or wherefore," but by simply waking up from the terrible nightmare of dualistic experience. If you are in a dark room, you do not ask why it is dark. You turn on a light and the darkness disappears.

When you have a headache you take it for granted that you have a head. Gaudapada would say: "What! You say you have a headache! My friend, you have no head!" He permitted no "erroneous" expression, none whatsoever. Sankara, on the other hand, would accept your erroneous statement, *i.e.,* "I have a head-ache," as a premise, and would then logically prove to you that the premise was wrong. He would say: "I will admit and accept their ravings, and then show them that they are wrong. Only One exists. Look closer, brother, not two—but One!" So Sankara accepts the erroneous statement that the universe exists, and then logically leads us to the acceptance of a Fundamental Reality.

This reminds me of something that happened in the life of Sri Ramakrishna. Once a devotee of his took a friend to see him at Dakshineswar. The man had just lost his eldest son and was half crazy because of it. He had not wanted to go to see a holy man. He had told his friend, "What use is there in going to see a holy man? He will just tell me that it is all illusion and that I should not be attached to my family. What good will that do me?" But the devotee had reassured him, saying, "This holy man is different. Come along with me."

Ramakrishna talked with the man about his bereavement. He listened to all he had to say. He asked questions about the son and sympathized with the man. He said he knew how he felt, because when his nephew had died he had felt as though his heart were being wrung as one wrings a wet towel. In recalling this, Ramakrishna's eyes filled with tears. The man, as well, was weeping. Together they wept for some time. The man was greatly relieved. Ramakrishna gradually worked a complete cure, and in the end jumped up and sang a heroic song, defying death. The man found peace. Ramakrishna was slow to work any changes. First he accepted the man's premises as true, as right, and then slowly brought him around. The man left in a consoled state of mind, relieved of his grief. Ramakrishna accepted what he knew was not truth and then led the man from there. In the end, the true nature of the son as the birthless, deathless *Atman* was established by Ramakrishna.

Sankarà expounded the *ajatavada,* or non-creation theory of Gaudapada, from the viewpoint of *vivartavada. When a thing has the appearance of being something that it is not*—that may be called *vivarta.* The classical illustration is that of a rope appearing as a snake. A traveller, passing through a village at dusk, saw a snake stretched across the road. He ran to the nearest house and cried, "There is a big snake on the road! Come and see it!" A man came out of the small house. "All right, let us see it," said the man. He picked up his lantern and started walking with the stranger to the side of the road. All the while the stranger was asking him such questions as, "What kind of a snake do you think it is? Is it poisonous? Are there many snakes around here?" To these questions the villager said nothing. As they reached the road, he moved the lantern down so the stranger could see clearly. When the light shone on the road, the snake turned out to be nothing but a thick piece of rope! This is *vivarta;* when something has the *appearance* of being what it is not.

On the other hand, the change of a phenomenon into something else, as milk into cheese, is known as *vikara.* Sankara takes a position between these two—*ajatavada* and *vikaravada.* He agrees that Brahman does not change. It remains the same. But, for some reason or other, it *appears* to change; not like milk into cheese, but rather as a rope appears to change into a snake. Therefore, Sankara expounded the vivarta, or *mayavada* theory, which proclaims that it is through or by maya, or illusion, that Brahman manifests itself. It is by the power of maya that the

One-without-a-second, Brahman, *appears* as the many. Sympatheti-cally, Sankara proposes the doctrine of maya, which makes non-existence existent. He says, in effect: "All right, I'll admit for the time being that the world is real—relatively real. It is as real as the snake superimposed on the rope is real. But when the light of awakened consciousness shines on this world, you will know it is not the snake. You will know its real nature."

To discriminate, to distinguish the real from the unreal—that is the theme of monism, or advaita, as interpreted by Sankaracharya. The real and the unreal have to be distinguished. "What sort of monism is that?" you may ask. Therein lies the distinction between the philosophy of Sankaracharya and that of his grand-guru, Gaudapada. Sankara assumes the existence of the unreal. Under the influence of maya we are bound to see duality. Sankara accepts this as a premise.

The *vivartavada*, or illusion theory, as expounded by San-karacharya classifies statements as *vyavaharika*, fact or relative truth, and *paramarthika*, fundamental truth. A fact is a reproduc-tion of a happening, while truth is that which never changes. A fact may not be true, but it is a fact because it has happened. Always try to distinguish between relative truth and fundamental truth. Try to understand these two aspects of any entity. See how a thing happens, go back to its cause, and when you analyze that cause you will know that only one reality, not many, exists.

The man in the rope-snake story did not answer any of the questions about the snake because he knew there was no snake. The snake-consciousness was illusion, maya. Maya is this: we see a snake where there is no snake. Where there is only One, we see many.

Sankara accepts the statements and experiences of people as vyavaharika, fact or relative truth, and logically leads them to the realization of paramarthika, or fundamental truth. Through logic give up vyavaharika. Then give up logic, give up every-thing! Logic is for enjoyment, not for liberation. Logic is within maya, too.

Brahman cannot be infinite, omnipresent and omniscient if anything else exists. Think it over. Man walks from one "truth" to another. All readings are relative. All readings of the final Truth are just readings. When the Absolute is realized, it trans-cends all operations.

Controversy, no doubt, consolidates one's opinion, and therefore it is good. Amidst all the good and the bad, avoid reaction. When you reach the top you will know that, good or bad, there is no difference. Both must be ousted. All is illusion.

To a strict monist projection never took place. There cannot be any maya. Where would it take place? There is nothing but Brahman. Sankara said: "How can I tell you what maya is? I take your statement *as* maya, and lead you right."

If you admit of anything outside the sole reality of Brahman, you are a dualist. Whether your Ideal be personal or impersonal, a God, force, or a Christ, you are a dualist. In fact, if you admit of any creation at all, you are a dualist. Sankara said that if you must know something about this world go to Kapila (the founder of the *Sankhya* philosophy with its *Purusha* and the twenty-four categories of evolution). As long as you are under the influence of maya, he said, go to Kapila if you want an explanation. Sankara taught that the world is maya or relative truth. It is a fact because it has happened, but it is not Truth and it has no real existence.

Sankara's school of monism remains supreme among schools of philosophy. He acknowledges mundane phenomena as "fact" and, instead of giving any final explanation of it (which he thinks impossible) he helps seekers advance from this relative world into the state of realization by means of discrimination and renunciation. These are the two watch-words of Sankara.

Sankaracharya summed up his whole philosophy in a very brief verse. "Whatever has been taught in thousands of books," he said, "I shall tell you in half a verse. *Brahma satyam; jagat mithya; Jiva Brahma eva naaparah!*" That is: "Brahman is the only reality; the world is unreal; the individualized soul, or self, is nothing but Brahman." These are the three truths that must be realized by a student following the path of jnana yoga.

Now there are certain qualifications necessary for one to become such a student: (1) human birth; (2) right understanding resulting in a strong desire to penetrate the mystery of life and death; and (3) close association of a liberated soul in the form of a guru.

In the attempt to manifest its potential power and perfection, the embodied soul must have experiences in various incarnations until it finally attains a human body. That affords it the highest opportunity to tear off the veil of maya, the cause of births and deaths. (The Hindu scriptures say that in order to be born as a human, the embodied soul has to pass through 8,400,000 incarnations in order to gather the necessary experiences in different stages of evolution!) You have the highest opportunity when born as man or woman, for only in the human body is it possible to apply the right method of discrimination. If you do not take advantage of this human incarnation, what an opportunity is lost to you! For now you can achieve the highest goal or be so degraded that you are born into a lower existence and forfeit, for the present, the right to eternal freedom. Your action in this life decides your next step. Therefore, having attained this valuable incarnation, let us strive always for discrimination,that we may grow to love the truth and cherish it more than the vanities of this world. Let us not waste this human birth.

The student on the path of jnana yoga aspires to realize truth by getting rid of maya and its grip. That is his problem. To seek a remedy for any problem one must have a thorough comprehension of its ingredients, and the implements necessary for its solution. This is the case, also, with the spiritual aspirant. Although he is taught from the very outset that all is maya, he has to *find this out for himself*. He does this by exercising discrimination between the real and the unreal.

This becomes easier of attainment if the student understands something of the nature of the human entity.

What do we know of the components of the human entity? How have things come into existence? What is the world's relationship to me? Thousands of years ago, the sage Kapila analyzed the constitution of the microcosm and the macrocosm; an analysis that still holds force today. Sankaracharya said that if we must explain this universe, we must go to Kapila. Well, in the beginning we must have some explanation. We cannot discriminate the real from the unreal unless we have some idea of what this "unreal" is composed of. We must know what we are dealing with.

According to Kapila, manifestation evolves out of the combination of two entities: Purusha, the efficient cause of the universe, the sentient principle, without expression; and *prakriti*, the substantial, material cause of the universe. We may say here that the cosmology of Kapila and the teachings of Vedanta differ mainly in that what Kapila called Purusha and prakriti, Vedanta describes differently and calls Brahman and maya. Vedanta refutes Kapila on two main points: the plurality of Purushas and the independent nature of prakriti. According to Vedanta, Purusha is one, not many. And prakriti is not the "substantial" cause of manifestation; there is no material cause, all is "immaterial." It is maya which is vivarta, or a superimposition on Brahman. Hence, it has no real existence apart from Brahman. That, briefly, is the difference between Kapila's cosmology and Vedanta regarding these two entities.

According to Kapila, prakriti, or maya, is made up of three potentialities, or qualities, called *gunas*. They are *tamas,* the veiling power, creating delusion and ignorance; *rajas* the projecting power, of the nature of outgoing activity; and *sattva,* the equilibrating power, giving rise in man to the desire to return to the Source of his being. According to Kapila, Purusha and prakriti, which has these three potentialities, combine and evolve into *mahat,* cosmic intelligence or universal undifferentiated consciousness; *ahamkara* or ego, 'I'-ness; *manas* or mind, the faculty of consciousness that swings, like a pendulum, between the two poles of certainty and doubt.

From the mind evolve the following: (1) On the objective side the five *tanmatras,* or subtle forms of sense objects (sound, touch, sight, taste and smell), which evolve into the five elements of ether, air, fire (light), water (liquid) and earth (solids). (2) On the subjective side, the ten senses, *i.e.,* the five active functions: expression (speech, thought-communication, etc.); reception or acceptance (the endeavour to bring anything within you); locomotion or the transference of the subtle, the mental or the gross body from one place to another; expulsion or excretion; and reproduction, a natural instinct in man for self-continuation. It is the urge for eternal existence.

The five passive functions of perception are hearing, touching, seeing, tasting and smelling. That, in brief, is the analysis of Kapila.

Now, the human being is composed of three "bodies" called *sariras,* meaning "that which changes." These three "bodies" are changeable; hence they are not the Reality, for Reality is not subject to change. Brahman, the reality within each one of us, is known as Atman. Atman is beyond these three bodies.

The first, outermost body is called the *sthula sarira.* It is the gross, material body, a tangible combination of the five gross elements. It consists of all the physiological and anatomical constituents of the body; namely, marrow (including the brain matter), bones, fat, flesh, skin, membranes, entrails, glands, nerves, veins, hair, nails, and the like. This outer body is sustained by food. The second sarira is the *sukshma sarira,* or the subtle body. It is contained within the physical body and uses the latter as its instrument of expression, just as a mechanic uses his tools. Hence, the subtle body is independent of the physical body as far as its existence is concerned, but it is dependent on it for its expression. It consists of fourteen members: *chitta,* or cosmic mind-stuff, the medium in which thought-waves, like sound-waves, or vibrations, are created and, in some cases, transmitted; *buddhi,* basic intelligence; *ahamkara,* ego-consciousness; *manas,* mind; the five *pranas,* or vital forces, and the five tanmatras, or subtle forms of matter.

The five pranas, or vital forces, are: (1) *prana,* the energy which draws anything closer to you, like inhaling air; (2) *samana,* the assimilating energy; (3) *apana,* the expelling energy; (4) *udana,* the uplifting energy; and (5) *vyana,* the equilibrating energy. The five tanmatras are the subtle material of the senses. Although the subtle body is subject to change, it is not as changeable as the material body.

The third body is called the *karana sarira,* or causal body, the innermost body. It contains the seed of avidya, ignorance of the reality. The consciousness of maya (of Brahman somehow appearing as many) has been planted in this body. The real Self, the Atman, is Brahman, which *seems* to be confined within these three bodies.

The Atman is also described as being within five covers or *Kosas. Panchakosa* means five sheaths, or receptacles, like the scabbard of a sword. A more modern illustration is of an electric light covered by five shades of different colours and designs. As we approach nearer the light, the shades become thinner and more transparent; the changes in colour and design represent the varying combinations of gunas or qualities. In order to reach the Atman within, we must eliminate these shades one by one through the power of discrimination.

The first and outermost cover is the *annamaya kosa.* It is the gross, material body (sthula sarira) which develops by means of food and decays without it. It is the grossest "crust" of the Atman. The second is the *pranamaya kosa,* the receptacle of vital energy, expressed through the organs of action. The third covering is the *manomaya kosa,* the receptacle of "mind." As the mental sheath, it consists of mind functioning through the five senses of perception: hearing, touching, seeing, tasting and smelling. The fourth sheath, or cover, is the *vijnanamaya kosa.* This is the perfect knowledge sheath where buddhi or intellect functions through the senses of perception. Thus we find that the second, third, and fourth kosas comprise the sukshma sarira, or subtle body. The fifth kosa is known as the blissful sheath. It is the causal body, or the karana sarira. It is the innermost "covering" of the Atman.

The five kosas may be thought of as five concentric circles with the Atman as their common centre. The Atman is at the centre of your being. What you have to do is to go towards the centre. Shift your "home" inwards. Discriminate, be introspective, contemplative, and then meditative. *It is the turning within that marks the beginning of the search for truth, for perfection.* Without that, no progress can be made. By exercising discrimination we move towards the Self. One by one, we must do away with the superimposition of these body-ideas which obscure our knowledge of the real Self.

In the waking state we "live" in the gross body. In the dream state our consciousness is withdrawn into the subtle body. In the state of dreamless sleep, consciousness is further withdrawn into the causal body. But throughout these three states of consciousness there is a continuity of awareness. When we awake from dreamless sleep, where we "knew" nothing, we find no break or change in our awareness. We pick up from where we were and go on. When we awake from deep sleep we know we are the same person who went to sleep. Now, how could this be true unless there was a continuity of self, a recorder of experience? How do you know that you were in the dreamless sleep state? Because it was recorded by Consciousness. The Atman is that Recorder, the Witness of all the changing experiences of the senses, mind, and ego, as well as the Witness of the absence of them (as in the case of deep sleep). In this state the Atman is separated completely from the agitations of the mind, senses, and ego.

The real Self of man exists independently of the sariras and kosas. The body, mind, intellect, ego, and all functions of the human entity, as well as the senses, sense-objects, and everything else cognized by the mind are known as non-Self, or maya. The

Atman is the Witness of all these. It is beyond mind, beyond all manifestations, beyond everything. It is changeless, eternal, aloof from motion, activity, and change. Our object is to realize That as our true self; but through the "interference" of maya we identify our self with the non-Self. It is simply a matter of false identification. We have to transfer the identification of our self, now firmly rooted in the body and mind, to Brahman.

Brahman is the All in all, and our constant endeavour must be to identify our self with That. The trouble is that we have the habit of identifying our self with the body and its functions. For instance, when we use the word "I" we have the idea of the body. At least 999 out of 1,000 think of the body as the "I." For that reason the limitations of the body are superimposed on the real Self, or the real "I." Do I have to prove it? If you ask a person how much he weighs he will put his body on a scale and perhaps say, "I weigh 145 pounds." If you ask his height, he will measure his body. He always ascribes the qualities of his body to his self. He accepts the qualities of a finite thing as his self, and yet expects to realize Infinity. What a contradiction! Is it possible? If you think you are the body how can you realize you are Brahman? How often do we use the expression "my body," and weigh it and call it our self. Why do we commit this blunder? I and my body are related as possessor and possessed. When you ask me how much I weigh I do not weigh my coat and say, "two pounds." Why should I do such a thing with my body?

We must understand the possessor-and-possessed relationship. Every perception involves two things : a subject which perceives and an object that is perceived. We say that we possess the body, mind, the faculties, and so on. We say, "My body, my head, my hand, my mind, my senses, my intellect." These are the perceived, not the perceiver. There should not be any confusion between subject and object in consciousness. Furthermore, the objects must always remain in the category of objects. If you have reached a conclusion as to what constitutes the objects, you cannot, the next minute, make them the subject.

Take the "I" and try to eliminate everything in the object category. As you analyze you will find that you *feel the presence* of the body, mind, and so on. In other words, the subject objectifies the body, mind and feelings. When I am angry I know I am angry. When I am happy I know it. Feelings, therefore, are nothing but objects in relation to the subject. If you can eliminate the body idea from the consciousness of the "I", you will have no reason to believe that the "I" occupies the space which is occupied by the body.

Why do we find it difficult to do this? Why can we not disentangle our self-consciousness from the body and its functions? Because a great power is obstructing us. A great power has created confusion in our understanding and, as a result, we are behaving as we are. Though "royal" descendants, we are behaving like beggars. Although we are Infinite, we think we are small, weak, and fragile.

Impelled by the power of maya we have reached this state of finiteness. We have forgotten our real nature. When this power of maya is understood we shall realize our true nature. Sometimes a glimpse of it comes to us like a streak of lightning, revealing the truth. But, just as lightning reveals a landscape for a brief second, and is then quickly covered by the darkness, the truth may be revealed to us and again seemingly lost. Of course, it is not blotted out from our consciousness altogether. It remains in much the same way as the consciousness of the landscape remains after that brief flash of lightning. The final state of realization, however, comes when the revealing "light" is retained fully and completely. To go back to our pristine glory, out of which we have been drawn by the power of maya, to attain that state and to remain in it, is to reach the final goal of jnana yoga—freedom.

It is very difficult to get out of this maya. It is indeed difficult to transcend our subject-object consciousness. All we understand is "I am *this*. I want to possess and enjoy *that*." Perhaps the idea of going to a heaven appeals to more people than the attainment of freedom. I remember that once Swami Turiyananda asked me a question abruptly when I went to see him. "Would you like to go to a heaven?" he asked.

I immediately replied, "No!"

He smiled and said, "That is because you do not believe there is a heaven. But suppose I can show you there is one? Then, would you say you would not want to go there?"

It is impossible for a mind that cherishes some desire, even the desire to go to a heaven, to appreciate the goal of jnana yoga. For it is only by denying dualism in all its forms that one can realize truth through the path of jnana yoga. On the lower plane, we must recall, there is always subject-object consciousness. We have to go beyond the mind. The mind is not constant; by nature it is fickle. What guarantee is there that the mind that today loves God or truth will not love the devil tomorrow? The "I" which associates itself with the mind must be removed. Only then will subject-object consciousness disappear. When that is gone the mind vanishes, and you realize your identity with Brahman. Thus nescience, or maya, is destroyed; its "veil" is removed once and for all.

When the superimposition of the mind upon the Self is done away with, then the bliss of Brahman is experienced. The mind's existence depends upon something else. It is "riding on the shoulders" of another! When its is submerged, drowned as it were, the bliss of the experience of Brahman is experienced. The control of the mind is the keystone that joins the two sides, phenomenal and noumenal, of the arch of maya. This arch must be pulled down.

Jnana yoga does not say that the realization of Brahman is to be "attained." It teaches no creed or ritual. It does not promise to give you anything you do not already have. Perfection is a state of unfoldment of consciousness; in that sense, it is not attainable. Perfection is potentially within you. As soon as the veil of maya is removed, *you become what you have always been.* The individualized soul, the jiva, is nothing but Brahman. Jiva *is* Brahman. The veil of ignorance that obscures this knowledge simply has to be removed. That is all.

2

THAT which you already have cannot be acquired, for you can never be without that which is your own. So it is said that Brahman cannot be attained. You *are* That at the present moment. But you have to realize it, you have to unfold this understanding of it in your consciousness. And that can be achieved by different degrees of intensity.

In the first place, you may achieve an intellectual conviction by hearing about it from a person who has, himself, gained that conviction. Such a person will discuss it with liveliness, vigour, and power. It is not to be got by reading books. It is a great privilege to be able to hear such a conviction from one who has demonstrated the truth of it in his own life, one who has gone beyond fear, beyond death, and beyond life (as we know it). Then, though you may not have actually realized it yourself, you no longer doubt it. You have gained a certain degree of "realization," an indirect knowledge of Brahman.

Do you realize that we have only indirect knowledge about many things we accept as true? How many have demonstrated to themselves the conclusions of science? Yet we accept these as truth and thoroughly make them a part of our accumulated knowledge. If we could once gain the conviction that "I am Brahman," even as mildly and indirectly as we gain conviction in other matters. it would revolutionize our whole life. We could no longer be the same persons. Not only that, we would find many misconceptions beginning to vanish.

It requires much practice and discrimination to transform an intellectual conviction into a real perception. Great spiritual teachers have, of course, encouraged us to work for *direct* perception of Brahman. That is the ideal. That is the goal. However. if, for the time being, we compromise, and first gain an intellectual conviction of the goal—but always holding to the idea that we will someday reach the final goal—we will make progress. The road leading to the final goal is very steep and slippery, and the pilgrim must be enquipped for the journey.

What is the difference between indirect knowledge and revelation? Suppose you enter a dark room. I also am in the room but know it thoroughly, and begin to describe it to you. I am describing everything in the room ; from this you begin to form concepts and gain a certain knowledge of the room. Then I turn on the light. What happens? You see the room clearly for yourself. Compare these two states of knowledge. When you first entered the room, before it was described to you, you might have thought many things—that it was an opium den, a thieves' hide-out, or some other such place. Then when you heard me describe it, you formed a better idea of it. You gained indirect knowledge of it. When the light was turned on you saw the room and verified my description. So it is with the knowledge of Brahman. Though you can gain indirect knowledge of Brahman, it is nothing compared with direct perception of it. Then all misconceptions and doubts vanish once and for all.

The individualized soul is Brahman: *jiva is Brahman. Tat Twam*

Asi (Thou art That) is the greatest of all statements. The student on the path of jnana yoga has to educate his mind to remove misconceptions that cling to it, those that make him think he is something else. In the last analysis, all that we need to educate ourselves in any field, material or spiritual, is discrimination—a kind of meditation to remove doubts—in order to realize the import of that one statement: *Thou art That.*

The buddhi and ego are liars! "I am so-and-so" is the greatest lie in the world. You are the Atman, the ever-free, ever-glorious Self, Brahman. You are the Witness of the buddhi and the ego and all their train of "followers." Know that nothing exists outside your real Self. Things, as they are perceived, are illusion, like a desert mirage. Are we then to walk about as if in a dream? No. In this mirage of the world let your body act, but with the *real you* inside serving as the Witness, knowing all the time that this objective world is not real. Have one set of teeth to scare people with, if necessary, but have your own private little set to eat with! In order to maintain this discrimination one must think a little.

In the West serious thinking is not emphasized. Activity has been glorified; *doing* is everything. But why brag about one's activity? Isn't it true that often the one furthest from the goal runs the fastest? For a change, cultivate a little inactivity, *inner* activity. Only then will you be able to appreciate spiritual life. You have extolled your shortcomings as virtues. This incessant activity of body and mind—has it brought you all you want? No. And it never will. The student of yoga must once and for all realize this. Then he will begin to question seriously the "why" and "wherefore" of things. The realization of Brahman is the only thing that will bring fullness and completion to your life. The zenith, the culmination of fulfilment is to be found only in the identification of your self with God, with Brahman.

"You are Brahman. Know that, and be perfect." Challenge this statement with logical objections and then find a solution within your heart, through an analytical thought process. Ask yourself: "If I am God, the Good, the True, the Omnipotent, why do I not know it?" You know that you are Brahman, intrinsically nothing but Brahman, but you will not heed it. You will not rid yourself of the delusion that makes you think otherwise. Why? First, because the reality has been "interfered" with by an *upadhi*. An upadhi means a limiting condition which makes a basic substance assume a different form from what it actually is. On the movie screen there are nothing but gradations of light. The film limits, or conditions, light. It is an upadhi. Space, on the other hand, is limitless but an enclosure gives the appearance of limitation. This apparently limiting condition is what is meant by an upadhi.

We limit our own understanding in reference to relative limitation. An upadhi may assume names and forms. A man makes clay models and says: "There is no more clay." He forgets that the clay remains, but it is now in the shape and form of the horses, elephants, tigers, and dogs he has modelled. Those shapes and forms are upadhis which have "interfered" with the clay.

This universe, known to us now through the different senses as a changing mass of objects, is in reality nothing but Brahman. There is no duality. When we speak of *this* or *that* we are only recognizing the forms, the upadhis. When we speak of *you* and *I* we are speaking of superimposed forms only. We have not realized the Substance, the Reality behind it all.

Second, we have been overcome by the power of maya. We are viewing this world, including ourselves, as the "snake" and not as the "rope". When the light of consciousness, freed from maya, shines on this world, you will know that it is not what you think it is. In other words, what we now call this world, with all its beings, with all its variety, is not actually real. Its reality is Brahman. Sankara says that we are like drunken men. Our viewing the universe as other than Brahman is the effect of the wine of maya. We must throw off that drunken delusion. That is the aim of jnana yoga, and it is accomplished by a qualified aspirant who follows the method laid down in this yoga.

Even if all the gods and goddesses appear before you, if the God in this temple, the God within, has not been realized, it will not help you to attain to the highest state. That great One within must be discovered. If you understand the goal, any method may be used to reach it. You must begin with the attitude that distinguishes the *I* and the *not-I*, the Self and the not-Self. When, by discrimination, you become established in the realization of the Self, the so-called non-Self merges into the Self and vanishes. Brahman alone remains.

It is not nothingness, but *all-thing-ness* that one attains through the realization of Brahman.

One realizes that: (1) Brahman is the only reality; (2) the universe of phenomena (as we know it) is unreal— its reality is Brahman; and (3) the reality of the individual soul, or jiva, is nothing but Brahman. Brahman is all that exists behind all the names and forms in the universe. It is a question of negation of the appearance, realization of the reality, of Brahman, and then affirmation of the presence of Brahman everywhere.

Then you will be able to say: "What I see is Brahman, fundamentally nothing but Brahman. Literally I see God everywhere." But you will know that you are not seeing Him as He is; you are seeing Him as He appears through these upadhis, these containers, these bodies and minds.

In the last analysis anyone who says, "I have not seen God" is a liar! You cannot see a thing without seeing God. It is a matter of conviction.

The jnani sees the same world as we all do, but he sees it in a different perspective. This universe is, in reality, nothing but Brahman. You are Brahman, present everywhere. You are one with the entire universe. Freedom, according to the jnani, means living in the awareness of Brahman at all times, under all circumstances.

The story is told of four sages who knew themselves to be Brahman. They went to visit Siva, the god of knowledge. They paid their respects to Siva and had a long conversation with him about the immortality of the soul. However, they did not notice that Yama, the king of death, was standing nearby. Yama was offended that they did not greet him. He decided to take revenge upon them. When they rose to depart he cursed them, saying: "Proud sages, you dare defy the king of death? I denounce you. You will have to take birth in animal bodies."

Yama is all-powerful over the body, so the bodies of the four sages were changed then and there into the forms of four dogs. Now Yama looked at them and said: "Do you see what I can do with you?" But the sages were illumined souls. They knew themselves to be bodiless, formless, sexless, all-knowing, omnipresent and full of bliss; so they did not feel any different. "Yama, you have no power over us. We are still Brahman."

Yama was very angry and transformed them into insects. But even as their bodies were changing they laughed at him. Yama felt insulted to find that the sages were unaffected by any change he made in their bodies.

At last Siva appeared before Yama and consoled him by saying: "Yama, you rule over those who know the body as their self. But those who know themselves to be the Atman, to be Brahman, are beyond your power. You may change the body, but what can you do with the real Self? You had best lest those four sages alone!"

Our consciousness, which is in reality perfect Consciousness, is now heavily burdened with many coverings. If we can eliminate these coverings that cling to this individual consciousness that we call "mine," call finite and imperfect, we will realize this consciousness as the perfect Brahman. When ignorance has been removed we find that we have all the time, always, and under all circumstaces, been and ever will be one and the same with Brahman.

Full and complete realization of that One is the goal and ideal of jnana yoga. We must not stop short of that goal. No idle talk; talking and quoting will not do. We must go beyond mere intellectual conviction and make it true perception. Of course, everyone does not have the same intensity. Most people would be satisfied with intellectual conviction. But if inspiration comes, if the flood gates open, if nothing else satisfies and one cannot think of anything else, cannot eat or sleep until he gains that direct perception, he cannot be satisfied with indirect knowledge. He will make every effort to reach the goal without delay. There are some who must be "express passengers"; others are not in such a hurry. Some people do not mind taking a slow train and looking leisurely out of the window at the passing scenes. Others are very much intent upon reaching their destination. If a thief knows that in a room next to him there are fabulous jewels he will not rest until he breaks through the wall and possesses them. If one has such intensity to realize Brahman he will strive constantly to remove the veil of maya, this wrong conception of himself. He will try to remove the concepts of body, mind, senses, and so on, which are so many superimpositions that seem to make the real Self smaller and smaller, that seem to limit it to this small container, the body and mind.

In our attempt to realize the truth, we must have great tenacity in our discrimination; for maya is always at our elbow! Maya covers individual consciousness with layers of obstructions.

These are layers we may look upon as types of energy known as tamas, rajas, and sattva. We have touched on these forces earlier, but they deserve further explanation. The first, tamas, is characterized by dullness of mind, inertia, inadvertence, ignorance, and laziness. Lust, anger, arrogance, envy, jealousy and other qualities born of an excessive sense of ego-importance are attributes of rajas. Sattva is expressed by such traits as absence of pride, faith, devotion to the search for truth, discrimination, and a strong yearning for liberation.

All of these characteristics exist in the human being. The effort of the student is to raise himself up to the state of sattva. He must throw off the lethargy of tamas and conquer the obstacles created for him by the power of rajas. The qualities of tamas and rajas will thwart all his endeavours at spiritual understanding. Those of sattva, however, will assist him until he gains enough strength to throw off the influence of maya entirely. The state of sattva is to be attained by effectively controlling tamasic tendencies and rising above the rajasic ones. Thereby, the student becomes ready for further instruction.

Some preliminary practices are essential for one who wishes to reach the spiritual goal. In fact, so important are they that yogis maintain these practices throughout their lives to keep their spiritual realizations intact. These practices have a deep and subtle application for those who are advanced in the practice of yoga; they are, as well, equally necessary for a beginner. Without practising these mental disciplines the mind cannot be brought to the state of sattva, in which the study of yoga is most effective.

There are five disciplines which, certainly in the beginning years, should be followed literally and uncompromisingly. They are: control of speech, non-receiving of gifts, entertaining of no hope, freedom from activity, and living in a secluded place. Sometimes, by broadening the scope of a practice we make it less intense. Let us first, then, narrow the scope and practise with intensity; then we may expand it. These disciplines help to curtail desires. It is desire that keeps the mind in a disturbed condition, dependent upon the external world for support; in fact, a slave to it. Can a slave be free?

Control of speech is very important. We do not realize how much disturbance speech creates in our mind. Practise the observance of silence for some time. You may start in a mechanical way at first, with gesticulations, pencil and pad. Later on you will find that you have no need for them. You will begin to control the *desire* to speak. You will think, "What do I care if so-and-so does not understand me? What does it matter?" Things that formerly seemed so important will retire and fade away. You will find this creation going on quite well without your conversation! Control of speech is essential to a quiet mind and an introspective one. Many people have maintained silence for long periods. Try it for a week. a day, or even a few hours each day. You will find many disturbing influences eliminated from your mind.

About *non-receiving of gifts,* be uncompromising. Say, "I do not want anything from anybody. I want to stand on my own feet. I do not stretch my hands before anyone. If I have needs, I shall pray to my own real Self for their fulfilment. I do not care for 'protection'. I let it go!" We must be able to stand absolutely alone and say, "I do not want anything but the Truth!" A time must come when we can stand like that, without props or supports. I call that the final realization of this discipline of non-receiving of gifts. When one has been able to feel like that sincerely, for a day, for a moment even, a great asset has been gained. A person who has come to that state has conquered desire. He does not need to seek things out; things seek him out.

The next is *non-entertainment of hope.* That creeper, hope—how it sprouts and grows and covers up everything! Relentlessly cut it down. Pull it out by the roots. That will give you immense strength. It is hope that weakens. The priests in the temple of a certain maharaja were very strong in their renunciation and the ruler began to feel uncomfortable about it, for they were a powerful influence in his kingdom. But the maharaja was a clever man. He thought: let me sow a seed of hope; so he said to them, "I find that all of you need better living conditions. Your stipends should be increased, and your food consist of more variety. I shall see to these things at once." A little seed planted! Gradually, the priests began to gather around the maharaja, anxious to please him. The seed began to sprout, and it grew and grew. The maharaja soon gained control of his priests.

In everything it is hope that binds us down and sucks our power. If you see God through a hopeful picture of heaven, you are gone! Hope will take you away from your main concern.

Why must we be slaves of hope? If you have hope as a motive force for work, you are a beggar. Hope is not a great asset for the accomplishment of anything. For a spiritual aspirant it is neither a necessary nor a good companion.

Freedom from activity has to be accomplished gradually. Why should we act? Action is an acknowledgement that we lack something. The more imperfect a person is the more active he will be. Activity betrays restlessness of the mind. Who is eager to act? One who has a restless mind, whose mind is not at peace, who has many desires. Rest from activity gives our constructive faculties an opportunity to function. Why should we work all the time? When are we going to enjoy our "pension"?

It is not possible to cultivate a spiritual mentality unless one *lives in a retired place* for some time. With the cessation of activities, in retirement, the contemplative faculty awakens and we begin to see things in a new and different way. We begin to understand the need to steady the mind and control the senses. It is very difficult to control the senses when we are surrounded by "Broadway"!* Solitude is necessary, especially in the beginning. Why should we follow the dictates of the senses and the roaming mind? Tell yourself: do I belong to them or they to me? If they belong to me they must obey me. But what am I doing? Obeying *them!* The mind cannot be steadied unless one has control over the senses. And, if there is always that environmental influence dragging the mind outwards through the senses, the mind will remain restless.

Retirement therefore is essential; even a synthetic retirement is better than none. If just now you cannot go into actual retirement practise mental retirement. Keep the mind aloof as far as possible from your activities. Daily feel that no one else lives in this world except yourself. Say: "I am the only resident in this world." That is a kind of meditation. Or for at least half an hour a day think that only God and you exist. You will come out of that half-hour "retirement" a different person. Even if you have to take up your busy life again that little bit of retirement will benefit you. Ramakrishna said: "Even after his bath the elephant will dip his trunk into a muddy pool and cover

---

*A term the Swami frequently used to denote a busy, worldly environment. [Ed.]

his body with that dirty water." The mind is like that, no doubt. But a little retirement is good even if the "elephant" of our mind gets involved with "muddy water" again. But gradually try to practise real retirement. Solitary meditation in real retirement gives one great courage even the courage to face death. I have experienced that courge when travelling all alone through hip-deep mud and water in flooded areas, while doing relief work. For a spiritual aspirant periods of retirement are absolutely necessary.

To sum up: control of speech is essential. Do not hanker for assistance of any sort or gifts of any kind from anybody. Stand alone. Have no hope, no plans . Cut away that creeper of hope. All these things weaken the mind and make it incapable of understanding the higher truths of spiritual life. Finally minimize your activity as much as possible and learn to love solitude. Actually go into retirement for some time. These preliminary practices will bring your mind to a state of steadiness and strength. You will feel less and less need for support from the external world. One has to be equipped mentally to take up the study of jnana yoga in real earnest. For one must be able to grasp the subtleties of deep spiritual truths. A gross-minded person will not in the least be able to understand what the practices of yoga are all about. Preparation is necessary.

<h1 style="text-align:center">3</h1>

A PERSON with the necessary qualifications or preparedness for following the path of jnana yoga may be described in Sanskrit as an *adhikari* meaning a student with a specific capacity. Such a person has developed the power to retain spiritual teachings. The practices we have just been discussing help the student to some extent to gain this competence. But there is more to it than that. There are certain other prerequisites that are essential for one to comprehend the teachings.

With reference to capability in spiritual life, people have been classified broadly into three groups: those who are fast asleep, those who are ready to be awakened, and those who are already awake. Naturally the vast majority fall into the first group and a very few would be considered as being in the last group. The sincere aspirant who has developed the necessary qualifications is known as the "ready to be awakened." Such a student may be called an adhikari.

There are several sources in Hindu literature where descriptions of the qualifications of an adhikari on the path of jnana yoga are mentioned. Manu, the ancient law-giver said that the aspirant should have gone through the three phase of life—*brahmacharya* [studentship], *garhasthya* [the life of a householder], and *vanaprastha* [retirement]—which are intended to lead one to the fourth stage of life, *sannyasa* [monkhood], which is the real quest for freedom. According to tradition, the aspirant should be at least fifty years old and finished with the first three stages of life. Ambitions and the so-called "preliminaries" of life should have been fulfilled. That is the idea. Taking to the pursuit of knowledge of the Self necessitates a great deal of renunciation; hence, it is said that a certain amount of futile activity should be experienced before taking up the path of jnana yoga. One must "tire out his wings." When you are tired of "fluttering," when a spiritual conviction has finally been reached, then you may discuss the "how" question in regard to the realization of the truth.

Scattered references are found throughout the Upanishads specifying that the adhikari must be *asishtha*, having great hope he will realize the truth. This does not mean ordinary hope. Fire yourself with the zeal of constructive hope. The adhikari must be *dradhishta*, or firm both physically and mentally. He must have *medha*, or brilliance of intellect.

The great saint and philosopher, Sankaracharya laid down very clearly the requisites necessary for an adhikari on the path of jnana yoga. These are known as *sadhana chatushtaya*, or the four-fold disciplines:

(1) *Viveka*, which means discrimination, discrimination between the real and the unreal; a firm conviction that Brahman is real and the universe is not.

(2) *Vairagya* or renunciation. Renunciation comes when one feels the urge to give up all transitory enjoyments, having understood their temporary nature.

(3) Possession of the so-called "six treasures":

Sama, which means calmness. Steadiness of mind is being able to hold the mind on the truth, after having detached it from the objects of the senses, knowing that they are transitory and therefore unreal.

Dama means self control: drawing within oneself the organs of knowledge and action and *holding* them within.

Uparati comes as a result of the practice of sama and dama. It is the condition of the mind in which it does not react to external objects.

Titiksha or forebearance, a state when the mind can maintain a calm and peaceful attitude under all circumstances.

Sraddha means firm faith, born of right judgment, in the teachings and also in the teacher.

Samadhana is self-settledness. It means the concentration of the mind that comes by constantly *affirming* the existence of Brahman.

(4) *Mumukshutvam* is the intense yearning for freedom.

These are called the four-fold disciplines prescribed by Sankaracharya. They have been defined and described in verses 19 to 27 of his great work, *The Crest Jewel of Discrimination (Vivekachudamani)*.

Knowledge is freedom. Though it does not depend upon any action, disciplines are necessary for the purification of ordinary consciousness. A stained or dusty mirror does not reflect the light before it. Our consciousness is like a mirror which, when cleansed and polished, will reflect the light of perfection, Brahman. The accomplishment of sadhana chatushtaya makes one a fit aspirant for the method of jnana yoga.

Viveka, discrimination, means the right appraisal of values. It is to be applied objectively and subjectively. In its objective application, it consists of right action, right judgment, right conduct. In its subjective application it is right self-analysis, right-mindedness, right attitude. By "right" is meant the action, or the judgment, that permits one to adhere to the fundamental principle of Oneness. Right judgment does not mean what someone thinks of it, or even what I think of it, but what it *is*.

Develop the faculty of discrimination. Realization is the prize you receive for your discrimination. Do not under-estimate the value of the prize. Do not think it is child's play.

It is in the nature of things to develop from the gross to the subtle. This is true of secular as well as spiritual knowledge. All knowledge is reached by moving from the gross to the subtle. I am reminded of a story. A teacher of astronomy was instructing one of his students. The conversation was something like this:

Teacher: Do you see that hillock in front of you?

Student: I do, Sir.

Teacher: Do you see a big tree standing on the top of the hillock?

Student: Yes, revered Sir. I see it.

Teacher: Do you see the branches of the tree?

Student: I see them, Sir.

Teacher: Do you see the topmost branch?

Student: Yes, Sir.

Teacher: Do you see a cluster of leaves at the tip of that branch?

Student: I do, Sir.

Teacher: Do you see an empty space in that cluster of leaves?

Student: I see it, Sir.

Teacher: Now, look closely at that space and tell me what you see.

Student: I see a star, Sir. A bright star.

Teacher: Good! Now, look just above that bright star and tell me what you see.

Student (after a few moments): I see—a—star, Sir. A very, very dim star.

Teacher: That is it! That is the *Arundhati* star!

That is a classic story called *Arundhati Darsana Nyaya*, which literally means "the process of showing the Arundhati," a small, almost invisible, star. It dramatizes the method of shifting the attention gradually from the gross to the subtle. The teacher leads the student's mind, taking advantage of the gross in order to reach the subtle. So it is with spiritual development. We must move from what we understand at the present to what we do not yet understand, from the gross to the subtle. We do this by discrimination.

It is nothing but egoism that separates us from Brahman. If we want to realize Brahman, we start the discriminating process with our lower self—the physical body with its attributes of hair, skin, fingernails, eyes—and then gradually penetrate deeper and deeper into the physical self until we grasp the ego. By eliminating the things we know we are not, we gradually draw closer to what we are. When we reach the ego we are quite near to the real Self.

Let us try to analyze this thing we call "self." I know I possess a body, so I cannot think I *am* the body (the possessor cannot be the same as the possessed). Who am I, then? Let us see. In this great realm of the body and inner faculties there is a king, so to say, who sits majestically on his throne. His subjects do not know how powerful he is. In fact, they are not even aware of his presence.

Now, let us imagine that there was a quarrel among the subjects of that king. "You do not do a thing worth mentioning," complained the legs and the hands to some of the others. "Look how hard we work! Just see how you, stomach, are pampered. You get everything nice to eat, but you do not work half as hard as we do! We're going to strike!" They were soon joined by some sympathizers. However after a time, they began to feel a bit weak. Just then a commanding voice was heard: "What's going on here? You menials have not even the power to end your own existence. Who do you think you are? It is *I* who hold you all together in order and harmony. It is only by my power that you are able to function at all. Don't you know me?"

They did not respond. "Well " he said, "Then I shall go!" And he started to depart. Then they all realized that without him they were helpless, incapable of any action. Without him their existence would cease. So, they gave up their strike and began to work together again. It is something like the presence of the boss in an office. .When the workers know he is present they stop talking and quarrelling and work quietly together.

The real "I" is like that king, always aloof, but empowering all operations of the mind and body. We must not allow the real Self to get mixed up with any of the "menials" who are merely rendering service for its benefit. By means of discrimination we have to meditate on this simile of master and servants right here in the kingdom of our body. For instance, what are the eyes doing? Bringing home to us colour, form, beauty. Is that for the benefit of the eyes? Consider this in regard to each of the senses and you will agree that the senses work solely for the benefit of the mind. The mind, however, is another servant, a sort of supervisor who sorts and organizes and puts things in their proper places. Now, for whose benefit are all these activities going on? As you proceed, discriminating along these lines, you will get a glimpse of the One who is beyond them all and who in no way shares the experiences of the members. He is the changeless Witness. Then you will understand that all changes, all dual perceptions such as joy, sorrow, and so on, belong only to the workers, the servants, not to the Witness, the real Self.

Imagine that you are standing on the balcony of your house. Below you, in the streets, you see a theft being committed and, shortly afterwards, someone performing some meritorious deed. Are you touched by either of these actions? If the police come and arrest the thief, are you responsible? If someone comes to reward the man for his deed, can you share in the reward? No. But you have been a witness to everything. Just so, knowledge proper (the real Self) is like a light within you that witnesses without taking any part in the actions that are going on in this complicated organism, the body and mind. Now I am talking to you. There is that Witness behind every operation of my body, mind, and intellect which radiates knowledge but does not take any part in their operation. Furthermore, it is only because of the presence of that Witness that the subordinate members can act. He holds, them all together as it were; he inspires them. But he, himself remains aloof and indifferent.

To realize that Witness as your real Self means to attain freedom, liberation, perfection. This is to be done by repeated discrimination. By means of discrimination we hold on to the real Self, the Observer, with our self-consciousness, and do not allow the Self to get mixed with the functioning of the faculties. This is discrimination. It has to be thoroughly and constantly practised. It is to be practised right here, within, by understanding this organism of the body and mental functions. If this superimposition of the non-Self on the Self, this mixing up, can be stopped freedom comes here and now. A saint is a saint; a man of realization is what he is because he has been able to establish within himself that discrimination more than other persons.

That great One within must be discovered. When we become firm in the realization of That, by discrimination, the socalled non-Self merges into the Self and vanishes. Then you realize the highest state of perfection. The veil of maya vanishes by itself when Brahman is realized. Maya is like a little girl who playfully says, "When I tell you who I am, I shall vanish!"

A senior Swami of our Order once posed a problem to some of us. It went like this: "Suppose you are the only person left on earth. Everything around you is turning into vapour, yet you still remain. What you call your body and mind are also gradually

G—4

vanishing. Think about it. Meditate upon it for seven days."
He was helping us to discriminate, to separate the non-Self from
the Self.

Thinking of the non-Self as the Self is the greatest of evils for
a jnani. This point must never be forgotten. By identifying
ourselves with the non-Self we leave ourselves open to all sorts of
agitations. These are the great obstructions, or enemies, to spiritual progress. But if we can withdraw, go within, into something more subtle, all those "enemies" will leave us alone.

This reminds me of a little story. A fox once said to a crocodile, "Look, human beings are great and powerful because they
cultivate the land. Let us do it also." They decided to raise
a crop of rice. The crocodile worked very hard, so the fox asked
him what he would like to take of the harvest—the root or the
top of the plant. "I think I'll take the root part as my share,"
said the crocodile. Next they raised sugarcane. This time the
crocodile thought he would fare better if he took the top part of
the plant. Finding that both times his choice was wrong, he said
to himself, "Certainly the fox has something over me. How does
he do it?" When he asked the fox, the fox said, "Oh, it is my
superior wisdom." "So, the crocodile's children were sent to
Mr. Fox to learn wisdom. Time passed, but the children did not
return. Mother Crocodile was anxious at the continued absence
of her children. She wanted to know how they were getting along.
"Don't worry, dear," said Father Crocodile, "they are getting an
education." However, the mother insisted; so the crocodile
went to bring his children home.

He found the fox swimming in a pool nearby his home, but
there was no sign of his children anywhere. He looked at the
fox suspiciously and asked, "Where are my children?" The fox
did not reply, but kept swimming happily in the pool. This infuria-
ted the crocodile. "What have you done with my children?"
he shouted. "I thought you were my friend! You must have
killed them, you wretch! Then I'll kill you. I'll eat you up."
He caught hold of the fox by the leg. "Eat me up?" laughed
the fox. "You have only caught my leg. You haven't caught
me!" So the crocodile caught the fox by his belly. The fox
laughed even louder. "You fool," he said, "that's only my belly.
If you can't catch *me*, how can you kill me?" The crocodile was
puzzled. He relinquished his hold, and the clever fox quickly

swam away from him. So Father Crocodile went sadly home, baffled at the superior wisdom of Mr. Fox. So we see that if we do not identify our Self with the non-Self, we can escape the grip of all our "enemies."

There was a man who was captured by some cannibals. They surrounded him in anticipation of a good meal. But the man took out his false teeth. Then he took off a false arm and removed his wooden leg. The cannibals were shocked. They cried in horror, "What can we do with him? He's just *parts!*" and they fled. If we treat our parts as parts (the non-Self as the non-Self) all the "cannibals" will be frightened away from us. We must discriminate between the Self and the non-Self and never confuse them. When we discriminate, we begin with two categories: the I and the not-I. Under the not-I is included everything we know in this world of phenomena. The "I" is the subject of the entire universe in which all things are objects. Every phenomenon in the universe is an object. Find out the subject. That is discrimination. To find out that real "I" is the very reason for our existence.

As the student progresses in the practice of jnana yoga, discrimination will take him deeper and deeper into the more subtle layers of his being. He will be able to withdraw his consciousness from the gross body and its activities, and then from the mental functions. Going further, he will recognize the ego (the cause of all the trouble) as the last superimposition covering the Self. Gradually that also will fall to his discriminative analysis, and he will at last stand face to face with the real Self and merge with it.

All this takes practice; and practice must begin with what we now understand, and then move on to what we do not yet understand. Begin your discrimination from this outermost layer, the gross body. Gradually you will be able to dive deep within your consciousness and discover your real Self, which is Brahman. Discrimination will guide you to the goal.

The accepted meaning of vairagya is renunciation. It implies strong dispassion and non-attachment. From vairagya arises true knowledge. With the attainment of that knowledge comes a natural withdrawal from the enticements of sense pleasures. This, in turn, results in the recognition of inner bliss, and what follows is peace.

One day a bird swooped down over a lake and caught a fish. There were many birds around the lake and as soon as he caught the fish they surrounded him, hoping to have a share of it. Wherever he flew they followed him. He felt very tormented. "How happy I was before I caught this fish," he said to himself. "But now these other birds are making my life miserable." He suddenly felt a surge of renunciation and dropped the fish. Immediately the fish was caught by another bird, who became the target of the others. The first bird, sitting quietly by the side of the lake, said to himself, "Now let them chase *him!* I'm through with it!"

Renunciation means remaining aloof and detached from everything. This detachment can be internal or external or both. When it is external, you have no object to call your own; no home, no family, no possessions. Nothing. And, what is more, you would not want them given to you. Though some people renounce externally, they still do not achieve their goal. Others renounce internally, but not externally. They may have every worldly object, but remain completely detached. Such people, of course, are rare. Then there are those who renounce both externally and internally. Siva is the highest example of that type. He calls nothing his own—a solitary yogi. The four directions are his clothes. He possesses nothing, yet he is the "Lord of the world." The practice of dispassion makes one fit for external and internal renunciation.

Now, let us suppose that we are all sincere students and have, by our discrimination, achieved a certain amount of understanding of Brahman. We believe that That alone exists and what we see about us is merely an appearance, or maya. What is our objective? It is to tear off the veil of maya. We must constantly try hard to feel that Brahman alone exists behind all the changing phenomena we experience. Trying to "see" Brahman in a person, we would very likely say, at first, "I do not see It. I see only a lump of flesh." We should struggle hard to eliminate the idea of that "lump of flesh." That is how we set about practising dispassion, by recognizing that what we see is not what we want to see. Through our repeated attempts at practising dispassion in this way, we may even develop an antagonistic, or even hateful, reaction to anything that obstructs the truth. I should not blame you if you wanted to tear off that veil of ignorance by sheer force. This attitude has been heightened by spiritual teachers when they have described the body as filthy, gross, and corpse-like; and when they have spoken of the universe as a snare which should be denied altogether. Such teachings are intended to make the mind of the student rebel against the nescience that covers the truth. They are intended to awaken within him a strong spirit of dispassion, leading him to renounce the unreal for the real.

If a person is enamoured of this body, an attitude of doubt should be created in him to "shake up" his consciousness. For instance, why *do* we think the body permanent? Because our conception of our self—that we are a man or woman, with a certain position in life, who possesses such and such things, and so on—seems to continue unchanged for some time. So we think the object of our conception is real. But if another set of experiences changes our present outlook, we would think this present state to be something false. We have five senses. Suppose that tomorrow we inherit a sixth sense? It would reveal a different world to us altogether. We now roam in the world of the five senses. With a sixth sense, our self-consciousness would undergo a complete change.

Now, we think that this body will take us across the great Ocean of the Unknown. We are floating on the Ocean of the Unknown and still we cling to this raft of the body, no matter how hopeless it may appear to us. We think: "I do not know where I have come from or where I am going, but with the help of this little raft I will get along *somehow!*" So we think. It is understandable that we may feel shocked when told this body is not permanent, is not real, is not at all what we thought it was. But if we patiently hear about the truth and try to understand it, we will gradually learn to correctly evaluate the body and its faculties, this little raft to which we cling so desperately! The endeavour of the spiritual teacher is to shock us out of our ignorance so that we may known our true Self. For that reason he helps us analyze our body, mind, and their functions. Thus, the student gradually develops dispassion for the temporary things of the world. Realizing that this little raft of his body and mind will not be able to take him to his goal, he begins the search for the real Self within.

The average man has no idea of the treasure that is hidden in this framework of the body and mind. He is so fascinated by this container, that it is very difficult to turn him inward. Let us suppose that one of your friends has a jewel box with a precious gem in it. But he does not know the jewel is there. He is hopelessly attached to the box and will argue that there is nothing else so wonderful. But you know the box has value only because of the jewel within it. Your friend's vision has been blurred by his inordinate attachment to the box; he is blind to anything else.

If you want him to know the truth, what procedure would you follow? It would be to shake his understanding, his evaluation, of the box. You might tell him, "Look here, you are raving about this box, but it has cracks in it. See? It is not as perfect as you think it is. And did you say it was made of real ivory? Oh, no, it is only imitation ivory." If you can create an attitude of questioning, of doubt, in his mind regarding the real value of the box, you will be doing him a great service. It is not you intention that he should hate the box, for that would be of no real benefit to him. Your intention is to make him realize the excellence of *something else* which he possesses but about which he is completely ignorant. So you criticize the object of his momentary adoration. That is what great spiritual teachers do for us. They point out the defects of the limited body and mind in order to teach us that we "possess" something of lasting value, something that will surely "take us across the great Ocean of the Unknown."

You cannot really give up. You cannot maintain an empty space. You get rid of one thing or one idea to make room for something better. You want to "bring in" Brahman, but all space is occupied. Instead, you must renounce certain ideas in order to "make room" for Brahman. Attachment to one thing is to be driven out by becoming attached to something else. As light enters a room, darkness vanishes. We simply have to let the light in. We must attach our self-consciousness to Brahman, to the Self, instead of to the senses, the ego, or the mind. To accomplish that, we must know the *value* of things. This leads to dispassion.

Self-consciousness must become joined to the Witness-self. The Witness-self is the one within us which watches without taking any active part in the operations of the body, feelings, senses, mind, intellect. When I am looking at you, for instance, I can feel that there is One within me that is watching. It knows but does not take any part in the activities of cognizing, analyzing, or understanding.

In every one of us there is this Entity that watches, as you can watch the activities of a marketplace from a high tower, the buying and selling going on below. You can see every detail from that tower; but you take no part in the activities. Similarly, there is an entity right here in your consciousness that remains aloof from all activities. You can feel it if you pay attention. It is watching everything that is going on in this body and mind—all your thoughts, feelings, and sensations. Sometimes you feel cold, sometimes hot; sometimes you are happy, sometimes displeased. But that One is neither elated nor displeased, not hot or cold. It simply witnesses these changing states. Very few people conceive, even intellectually, that such an entity is right there, in their consciousness. But it is there.

That Witness does not participate in any operation of our being. It simply watches. Think of it watching the mind. What is the mind doing? Let us look upon the mind as a travelling salesman who goes from door to door, concerned about little losses and gains. Sometimes he knocks at the door of Mr. Colour, sometimes at the door of Mrs. Taste, or Miss Touch. Is it not so? If you watch the mind you will find that this salesman is constantly knocking at the doors of its five good customers—Touch, Taste, Hearing, Smell and Sight. The mind is always busy contacting these customers and in this way the larger part of its power and strength is consumed.

Can this salesman go on constantly buying and selling? Does he never get tired? Has he no home? Ask your mind, which is always going out knocking at the doors of the senses if it does not want to come home and rest. Surely it will answer, "Yes." It does want to go home, but it is being goaded again and again to go into the busy market place. Let it come home! Allow the poor mind to come home. Let it throw off its bundles of wares and enjoy some rest and peace.

Now, how does the mind learn to come home? It hears a call, a call from within. The call is always coming from within, but most of the time it is drowned in the din and bustle of the marketplace of this world. It is lost in that noise. But there comes a time when the mind catches a faint echo of that call, and the clamour of the marketplace subsides for a while. That call inspires the mind; it begins to feel an urge to return to its home. It thinks, "What am I doing here, picking up a few pennies, while I have a treasure waiting for me at home?" This call produces no feelings of disgust or sense of defeat. Rather, there is so much attraction to that voice that it overpowers the desire for activity. When the mind hears the clear and lingering note of that divine call from within, it gladly turns towards it. It gladly turns away from the doors of its customers. It then realizes that nothing of any permanent value can be gained by all that activity. It feels that it *must* go home. And the mind's home is in the depth of our consciousness.

This is when the spirit of dispassion develops within us. But remember: dispassion does not mean hatred for this "unreal" world. When one knows with a sure and calm understanding that nothing much can be gained by trading with the objects of the senses, one does not become a pessimist. He may still meet sense objects but he does so with a profound sense of indifference. Not a shallow sense of indifference, not hatred. When you expect much from sense objects, disappointment is bound to result. When you expect nothing, then a contact is simply a contact —a matter of fact. You may still confront phenomena, you may still have to exist in the marketplace of life, but you are a merchant who knows the truth, who lives out his allotted span knowing it to be just a pastime. Your contact with colour, touch, smell, and so on produces no reaction. Do you understand? *You* are always aloof from action.

Both discrimination and dispassion contribute to an understanding of the true nature of the Self. You may gain some understanding of the Self during an hour's discussion; but when you go home, you become unsettled about it. You seem to gain something, only to lose it. A certain weed grows over ponds in India and covers the whole surface of the water with a sort of film. But underneath, the water remains cool and clean. If you want to drink the water you must push the film away. But as soon as you remove your hand, the film returns. Discussion about the Self, hearing about it, reading about it, contemplating it, creates such an opening in the mind. But the opening is soon covered by other things. Broadly, speaking, these are passion and attachment. Attachment is the clinging of self-consciousness to the body and its functions, to the mind and the ego. Passion exists when a certain object creates agitation in the mind. If our relation with the world, with our environment, is coloured by attachment and passion, the "weeds" rapidly cover up the opening made in the mind by our spiritual practices.

Discrimination and dispassion are the fundamental requisites for the attainment of the goal of jnana yoga. Dispassion, however, must be balanced and reinforced by a pure realization of the Self. Sometimes dispassion has been practised by ascetics with a passion! Though their goal is to be free from passion, they fear it so much that they passionately strive to become dispassionate! This is a type of reaction. Dispassion is a discipline that must be cultivated by knowing the right value of things. Dispassion and discrimination go hand in hand, and must work in harmony. They are like the two wings of the bird of renunciation without which it could not fly.

Sama and the other five requisities are known as the "six treasures." They may also be called the "six-pointed star." If this star is shining in the heart and mind of the aspirant it makes the yearning for freedom, mumukshutvam, possible. Without the possession of these requisites there can be no desire for real freedom. Sama has been described as resting the mind on Brahman after having attained calmness, which comes as a result of detaching the mind from sense-objects, knowing their defects. For the primary defect of sense-objects is their ephemerality; therefore, they cannot lead to the realization of Brahman.

How can we attain the necessary detachment? By controlling the outgoing tendency of the mind. There are two tendencies of the mind: outgoing and incoming. Usually the mind, pulled by the senses, rushes outwards. But it can be trained to go inwards. If you think about it, you will see that the senses, like so many wild, wayward children, are taking every opportunity to rush outwards, dragging the mind with them. But after many such experiences, the mind begins to understand that nothing of a permanent nature can be found in this way. Then it becomes satisfied, resting within; calmness comes to it. It is not being dragged here and there by the senses. As you grow to appreciate inner calmness, attachment for outer things naturally diminishes. You will then find nothing wrong with an expression like, "this corpse-like, filthy, impure body." To have such a reaction is, in itself, a great achievement.

Dama has been described as self-control. It means the control of both, the organs of knowledge (the eyes, ears, and so on) and the organs of action—the vocal organs, feet, hands, etc. Technically, dama means not only the control of these but the settling of them in their "respective centres". That is to resolve them into their subtle causes, or source. Its fullest intention is the complete cessation of all thought and action.

Consciousness must be detached, step by step, from the gross body, the senses, the mind, the buddhi and the ego. This is first to be done by controlling the outgoing tendencies, and later by resolving the inner faculties into their source. This results in self-withdrawal, or uparati. It is the state of consciousness when the mind, drawn within and made calm and steady by the practice of sama and dama, does not react to external objects or impressions.

The great Swami Turiyananda, a direct disciple of Sri Rama-krishna and a man of the highest realization, once underwent a very painful operation. He remained conscious throughout, and calmly watched the whole of the operation. Later he said, "I saw it as something outside myself. Therefore, I suffered no pain whatsoever." He was a great yogi, so he could do that.

We must begin by "keeping the mind at home," so that it does not exercise itself on sense stimuli in any way. Be able to dictate a few emphatic "No's" to the mind. Deprive it of its pet toys, the senses and sense objects. This is a great generator of power. It has to be experienced. It is difficult to convince you by mere words. At present, the mind, with the senses, projects itself outwards. It has not been taught to stay within. In fact, most people would feel very miserable and lonesome if they could not contact the world of the senses every moment of their waking life. They do not know that within them is something that will give them greater satisfaction.

First we must put a fence around the senses and pull them within. When we have silenced the mind and the inner faculties, the memory and so on, only the contemplative faculty remains. We must then bring the mind into the buddhi—no more contemplation, no more thinking of the *pros* and *cons* of things. We must just feel the *presence* of something within. When you are visualizing the image of, say, your highest spiritual Ideal, you are not thinking. Just the presence is there. But there is still subject-object consciousness. Something is seeing (visualizing) something; but there is One that sees both. Your buddhi is aware of something, but *You* are the witness of both the buddhi and that "something." The three disciplines of sama, dama and uparati, if steadily and sincerely practised, will bring us to the point where real meditation begins.

Titiksha means bearing all afflictions without trying to redress them, and being free from anxiety and lament. A character that has not learned the lesson of forebearance is very changeable, very whimsical. A character should be well-ground, well-chiselled, to fit the die of titiksha. Titiksha is the character-building discipline. One must be able to bear hardships in order to proceed happily in any field of life. Forbearance makes for a better person in any role. Remain unperturbed and forbearing in all experiences. Learn to endure the rigours of external nature for the fulfilment of internal nature. This makes one more tolerant, more broad-minded. Titiksha, the great character-builder, makes one dependable, loyal, steadfast, more sensitive; more loving, and more universal in outlook. It sharpens all the faculties. It makes one able to stay beyond the "pairs of opposites."

We have to practise titiksha in order to counteract our inability to adapt ourselves, without complaining, to different environments. This brings us great strength. Always remember titiksha, the character-building discipline.

Sraddha means faith and confidence, both subjective and objective. It means confidence in the external sources from which one expects help, including faith in the teachings and the teacher. It also means faith in one's self. It is not to be confused with foolish optimism. It is confidence built upon correct judgment. Know that the capacity to accomplish things is within you. If you want to do a thing, you can do it. But do not be foolhardy. Maintain a steady, calm, sober, discriminating consciousness. Select your associates with discrimination. They are bound to influence you, so choose them carefully.

Never for a moment think that you are weak or insignificant. Understand this, once and for all time: if you think yourself weak and helpless, if you are disappointed in the way you express yourself, do not come to the conclusion that divinity is not within you. *It is there.* It can never be dimmed or extinguished by any power on earth. Repeat to yourself: "I am divine. Divine perfection is within me." Repeat "*I am divine perfection*" ten thousand times a day.

The germ—the potentiality—of whatever we want to become is within us. We have to be convinced that the Ideal exists within and then work hard to remove the obstacles by our own efforts, not depending upon any individual or organization. Then alone does the Ideal become a part of ourselves. Moreover, we *know we are It.* It is not a question of acquisition at all. A painter, an actor, a singer, a doctor, a lawyer, or a spiritual man—each must work, discriminate and meditate to realize the truth, fully and completely, that *he is That.* He expresses himself with perfection in proportion to his realization of his identity with his Ideal. First, gain the conviction that divine perfection is within you and then do something to drive that conviction deeper and deeper into your consciousness. Be inspired with the Ideal; feel that it is already within you, ready to unfold. And with that conviction, analyze yourself closely. Find out all the obstacles within (not outside) you and then do something to remove them.

If obstructions come your way, say, "I am going to knock them down!" Do not fear obstructions. Strike at them. Circumstances will yield to you when you exert your strength to conquer them. There are four essential things necessary for a student in any path. I call them the Four S's: Strength, Steadiness, Simplicity, and Sincerity. Develop these within yourself.

Cut your bonds and come out! If you are down, do not despair. Kick the ground! Never let it be your friend. Inspire yourself with the confidence that whatever you want to attain is not something foreign to you. It does not have to be transplanted in you. It is a birthright you carry always within. Such confidence, Sraddha, is half the achievement.

Samadhana mens steadfast concentration on the Self within. This involves determination, fixity of purpose, one-pointedness. Let God-realization be your goal in life. Link everything with that highest goal or ideal. Let every occupation be regulated in harmony with that. "I live for God-realization; I live for the realization of Self." Stick to that statement throughout life.

Mumukshutvam means intense desire for freedom, for liberation; not only the desire for freedom, but a "passion" for it. The appreciation and attainment of freedom is the greatest thing in life—freedom, non-dependence on any sense faculty or circumstance of life! In a state of freedom, the centre of happiness is built nowhere; for that reason it is everywhere. Love of freedom includes the love of freedom for others also. Passion for freedom is expressed in an eagerness to remove obstacles in the paths of others, as well as in your own. Do not think of freedom only for yourself. Remember, all people are seeking freedom in various, and sometimes devious, ways. But everyone, consciously or unconsciously, is seeking it. The conscious love of freedom is a great virtue that expands the heart and understanding. Never impose anything upon another. Always respect his freedom. You are nothing but Brahman seen through a "container." The freedom of the soul *appears* to be interfered with by superimposed qualities, which are called upadhis. Space, for instance, is limitless; but we put up partitions and rename it as a room, a box, or some other container. However, it is nothing but space "contained" within certain limits by the partition or upadhi. Similarly, you are nothing but Brahman limited by the container of body, mind, ego, and so on. Imagine an infinite expanse of ocean, with glass bottles immersed in it. Within that ocean we, like glass containers, are moving about, filled with the water of the ocean. The water appears to be the colour of the containers because we are seeing the substance through the different bottles. But the water is colourless. That infinite ocean is Brahman, which is filling up each one of us.

Now what is the purpose of all these bottles? As they move about, up and down, to and fro, one bottle may look at another and think, "I'd like to be like that—a big bottle!" So it evolves, and experiences what it wants. After going through such a process over and over again it at last develops the attitude: "I do not want to be a bottle any more. I want to be the ocean!" No matter what the size of the bottle, it is now too small. It wants to be the ocean. That is mumukshutvam. That is the real desire for freedom, for liberation from all bondage.

By the intensity of mumukshutvam, a force is stirred within you. An affinity is created, and your feet are guided to a guru. It is said that a guru finds his disciple and not the reverse. But the *longing for freedom,* mumukshutvam, puts you in the right state of readiness. Then the guru appears. So, it is said in the scriptures that the aspirant, "being firmly fixed in the fourfold disciplines, approaches the guru with faith, humility and reverence, who leads him to the realization of the Self."

In the final analysis, there is no need for a human guru. But, because of lack of understanding, confusion of thinking, and various other obstacles to the realization of the Divine within, a guru is necessary for the attainment of the goal. A candle has the potentiality of light but it must be kindled. Man has the potentiality of perfection. It must be "unveiled" by the gurus' "kindling" of the inner potentiality.

4

THERE are two types of gurus. There is the *satguru* who gives the disciple *diksha,* or initiation. He can be only one. Then there are the *upagurus,* who may be many. Persons from whom we learn anything may be called upagurus.

What are the signs of a real spiritual guru? First, he is one who has himself gone through all the disciplines and has realized the truth. Second, he is one who is learned. That does not mean that he is one who can glibly quote scriptures and deliver orations, using all the available high-sounding philosophical terms. He need not have encyclopaedic knowledge; rather, he must be balanced in his learning in both the theoretical and practical sides of the science of the Spirit. His ethical, intellectual, and spiritual life must be in balance.

Third, he is one who works without any selfish motive, such as for money, fame, or the desire for leadership. Those great souls who may be called real gurus plainly show in their lives a disregard for all these things.

Fourth, a real guru is one whose love for suffering humanity "flows like the warmth of the spring season." Spring comes to all, indiscriminately. The person himself determines its influence.

Once a devotee went to visit Sri Ramakrishna at Dakshineswar along with some friends. After a short while the friends became restless. They began to whisper among themselves, "When shall we leave here?" Seeing that the devotee was not planning to leave soon, they went to the boat to await for him. Those boys were unable to absorb anything of what that Godman, Ramakrishna, was so lavishly dispensing to all around him. Those who are ready can benefit by the great gurus; others cannot.

Satgurus are classified as *Isvarkotis* (the divine category) and *jivakotis* (the human category). The Iswarkoti can take on complete power of attorney for a *sishya,* a qualified disciple, and give him full illumination regardless of the latter's own efforts. The jivakoti shows the path and encourages the disciple to follow it, and the latter must follow it in order to realize the goal.

The signs of a real sishya are:

1. Sincerity of purpose. He must want nothing but the Truth.
2. Steadiness in sadhana chatushtaya, the four disciplines.
3. Steadiness of will. He must be strong and healthy.
4. Sharpness of intellect. He must be full of hope and fervour.

It is steadiness and perseverance that lead to the goal. Steadiness followed by "inwardness" has been emphasized over and over again by all the teachers of yoga. Do you practise something every day? Do you *do* something? If so, you are steady in your intention and have sincerity of purpose, your practice will lead you towards higher and higher stages of realization. The sheer force of sincere practice will bring you the desired prize of illumination.

Cultivate "inwardness." Do not run after any sense object without questioning it carefully. Remember: "all that glitters is not gold."

When the mind wants to go outwards, ask it: "What do you want to go out for? Do you want to find in the world the beauty that never fades? I will put you, mind, in touch with the Supreme Beauty. Do you want to contact something that will quench your thirst, your desires, forever? Then turn towards the Infinite. There is no satisfaction in the finite. The happiness of the finite is not lasting, it has an end."

In this way, by cultivating the power of discrimination, you can turn the tide of the mind inwards, towards the attainment of the highest spiritual perfection. In fact, it is only when you get a glimpse of the internal beauty of the divine Self that you will never again be enslaved by the external world.

When one gets a taste of the realization of that inner Bliss, what does one care for outer things? When one has heard the music of divine musicians, can one be enchanted any more by the songs of sirens?

The spiritual current of inwardness helps him develop such an atmosphere around him that he attracts spiritual force to him. By such spiritual affinity he draws toward himself spiritually advanced people. There is no more powerful agent for the advancement of a soul than spiritual companionship. It is by this force of affinity that the aspirant meets his guru. Then his success is assured.

I am reminded of a beautiful simile. A little boat, drifting and tossing about on the ocean, is picked up by a big ocean liner and tied fast to it. The liner can cross the ocean with ease. By itself, the little boat has not the power to withstand the waves and the storm and to cross the ocean alone, but when tied to the larger ship there is no more danger of its being lost. It is that contact with the big ocean liner that brings security to the helpless little boat. Similarly, the safety and success of the pilgrim in spiritual life is assured as soon as he contacts his guru. Says a Hindu poet: "Make yourself ready to be attached to that great ocean liner of spiritual force (the guru) and you will easily cross the ocean of life."

If you were to ask, "How do I find a guru?" I should say that the safest way is not to try to find one at all, but to attract a real guru by becoming fit to be a real disciple. When you attract a real guru you know it; there cannot be any doubt about it. And the relationship lasts through eternity. In the whole range of human experience there is no relationship between two human souls so grand, so magnificent, as the relation of guru and disciple.

The teacher-student relationship between a satguru and a sishya is described in this manner: The satguru is like a lighted torch which brings out the potential fire in the sishya. The disciple is waiting to be touched by the guru in order to manifest the fire within him. The qualified disciple is like a dry piece of wood containing potential fire. But he cannot manifest it until he is "kindled" by the guru.

The guru inspires the sishya by his example, and he purifies him with his teachings.

The medium between the guru and the disciple must be unobstructed love on the part of the guru. This bridge must be there or there can be no conveyance. When this golden bridge is established, the communication begins.

The method of instruction proceeds through three stages: *Sravana, manana,* and *nididhyasana.* Sravana literally means "hearing," the process of "taking in." The guru teaches the disciple to "hear" the truth. The guru expresses the truth and the disciple receives it. This is a repeated process. Do not think that by hearing it once or twice the hearing process has been finished. There are many obstacles to the understanding of the teachings. Sravana means both hearing and retaining what one has heard.

I am reminded of an old folk story. There was an old demon named Vikata. All his life he had been killing human beings as men kill mosquitoes. Now he was tired of such an easy game. He decided to add some zest to it. He said, "I'll give them a chance to win!" Near his mountain home there was a huge pile of skulls of people he had devoured. He went out to it and picked up, very carefully, four skulls, saying to himself, "Ah, yes, I remember you all."

He put the skulls in his bag and went down to a nearby village. He sat down and laid the four skulls out before him. Of those who passed that way he asked, pointing to the skulls, "Which of these men was the wisest?" No one could answer. The very sight of the demon and the skulls sent a chill through them all. Vikata said, "No answer?" So he seized them and put them into his bag. This went on for a couple of days.

The villagers did not know how to protect themselves against this menace. They sent word to a holy man who lived in the next village. Early the next morning he came. He approached Vikata and said, "What are you doing here?"

Vikata said, "All my life I have devoured every human being I wanted. Now, in my old age, I have found a way to make it more interesting. I play a game with them, and give them a chance to win."

"What is the game?" asked the holy man. The demon replied, "I simply ask them which of these four men was the wisest. If they cannot answer, they are mine. Suppose I ask you the question. What would be your answer?"

"Just a minute," said the holy man. "What if I *do* answer your question correctly?"

"Oh," said the demon, "I hadn't thought of that. Well in that case, I shall surrender my power to you. I play fair!"

"All right," the holy man said, "If I can answer the question you must reform yourself and give up this terrible business of eating people!"

The holy man picked up one skull, looked at it carefully, and dropped a little pebble into one ear hole. The stone passed through the skull and fell out of the opposite ear hole. Laying it aside the holy man said, "A foolish man was he. Words of wisdom entered one ear and left through the other, without so much as touching anything between!"

G—5

He picked up another skull. When he dropped the pebble into the ear hole of this one, it fell out through the mouth. "Well do I know this kind of man," sighed the holy man. "Wise counsel he sought, indeed, but only to waste it in idle prattle. The mouth spent faster than the ear heard, leaving him always in poverty."

He reached for the third skull. Vikata, the man-eating monster, watched with both fear and fascination. The holy man dropped the pebble into the third skull and from the ear it found its way out through the throat. "He was a good man," said the holy one, "but weak. Receiving knowledge he enjoyed the taste of it. But he never tried to use it, to follow it in his life. He put off until tomorrow. But tomorrow never came!"

When the stone was dropped into the fourth skull it never came out! "A truly wise man was he," said the holy man. "He kept wisdom always within. Whatever he learned he retained, and his whole life was guided by that knowledge."

Vikata, a man—or monster—of his word, said, "It is my good fortune to have been defeated by so great a man as you. In my next life may I have even an ounce of your power! My life is yours, sir."

The holy man smiled and said, "I do not destroy. I build, even on a foundation of ruins. If you can follow the way of the fourth man, I will teach you the path of wisdom."

Vikata became a disciple of the holy man and whatever went in his ear never came out of his head. He grew to be a great sage.

This is a very instructive little story. The secret of success in any endeavour is to be able to retain the teachings, to assimilate them, and to make them one's own—to *live* and *be* what you believe.

So, sravana, or hearing, is the first stage in receiving the instructions given by the guru. The disciple must first hear, with sraddha. After hearing the truths expressed and explained by the guru he comes to the next stage of manana.

Manana means argumentative assimilation; it signifies the action of the mind when it swings between doubt and certainty. When the mind is considering a proposition it swings between these two poles, like a pendulum. The student raises arguments not to show off his "learning," but to understand the truth. It is a process of agitation, fermentation . As the result of manana the mind gradually becomes contemplative, and finally demonstrative comprehension of the truth is gained.

Let me give you a little story as an illustration of manana. A student of philosophy was studying at home when his wife asked him to go to the oil man for a bottle of oil for the lamps. On his way to the house of the oil man, he was continually thinking of his study. He was introspective. While waiting for the oil man to give him the oil, he noticed that the oil mill was run by a bull. The bull was blindfolded and was walking round and round grinding the oil from the oil seeds. Though the oil man was busy with his customers, he always knew when the bull stopped walking because he had put a string of bells around the bull's neck. When the sound of the bells stopped the oil man knew the bull had stopped, and he goaded the animal on.

The student of philosophy said to the oil man, "Oil man, you certainly are very clever. You would have made a fine logician!" Well, he took his oil and started home with it, still enwrapped in his admiration for the oil man's logic. "The walking of the bull is co-existent with the ringing of the bells," he said to himself. "When the bull stops, the sound of the bells stops. Very clever!"

As he proceeded down the road towards home he began to wonder if there could be any flaw in the oil man's logic. "The walking of the bull is co-existent with the ringing of the bells.'² He turned this over and over in his mind. Suddenly he threw down the bottle of oil and ran back to the oil man. "I've got it! I've got it!" he shouted.

"Got what?" asked the bewildered oil man.

"I've found the flaw in your logic! Oil man," he said, "suppose your bull stops walking, and stands still and *shakes his head!* The sound of the bells is *not* co-existent with the walking of the bull. See?"

"All I can say," said the oil man, "is thank God, my bull didn't study logic!"

So we see how first the student accepted the premise and argued it in his mind. When he found a flaw he went back to demonstrate it. His manana resulted in demonstrative comprehension of the truth of the proposition.

Nididhyasana literally means "meditation towards"; when meditation becomes constant and automatic, like the constant flow of a liquid. Nididhyasana is a constant and spontaneous flow of knowledge. The thing learned becomes your own. becomes a part of yourself. *You know you are it.*

To take a simple illustration of the three steps in the unfoldment of knowledge, which may be applied to any system of education: Suppose you teach a small child the word "good." He hears it (first step), but to him it is only sound and, therefore, he may forget it quickly. On his being commended as a "good" boy the word comes to have some meaning for him (second step), and he is good at various time. Perhaps, "good" at last reveals its complete meaning to him and he perfects himself so that "good" is always present as a part of his personality (third step). He *becomes it.* Many people gain the first two steps but do not reach the third one. They do not *become* what they believe. They live dual lives, believing one thing and doing another.

The student of jnana yoga has to exercise the powers of sravana, manana, and nididhyasana to realize the truth regarding the nature of Brahman, this world of phenomena, and of his own self. The formula has been set forth by Sankaracharya in these three statements: (1) Brahman is the only reality. (2) The universe of phenomena is unreal. (3) The human soul, or self, is nothing but Brahman. The student hears the truth of this from his teacher, who quotes from the scriptures and from men of realization. He may speak from his own experience; he may use similes and metaphors pertaining to contemporary life in order to "drive home" the message to the student. The teacher emphasizes the importance of the teachings in every way; by repetition and reiteration he instructs the disciple in the truths to be realized.

The student hears the teachings and contemplates them with attention and with the faith that he will be able to understand and realize them. And he analyses them within his mind in order to assimilate their truth. He meditates upon the teachings and strives to remove the ignorance surrounding the true nature of Brahman, the world, and his own self.

Concentration—constant thinking on the Ideal—has been prescribed as the means to bring about that realization. What we concentrate upon, we become. If we concentrate upon Brahman, the truth, we shall become Brahman. But it is a gradual process. One illustration is of a hornet catching a small roach. Though the hornet stings his victim, he does not kill him. The roach is numbed, loses its senses, and the hornet carries it off to its nest.

There it lies in fear for awhile, concentrated only on the hornet. Gradually, a metamorphosis takes place. The insect is changed into the form of a hornet; there is very little difference between the two. This has been seen by many people. If, however, you feel reticent in accepting this illustration literally, you will find many others in modern psychology. Thought forms the physical structure, the make-up of an individual. In fact, we may say that physical expression is nothing but the manifestation of thought within an individual. If you think mean, ugly thoughts you will become mean and ugly. The reverse is also true. Now, if you start concentrating on the fact that you are the perfect, immortal, Absolute Being within, that Being will gradually be reflected on your consciousness. Of course, the individual consciousness cannot reflect That completely, but the "metamorphosis" will slowly begin to take place.

To become absorbed with the thought of the Divine within us is, of course, a figure of speech. Brahman is not located in any space within us. Brahman is like the ocean and we, like so many containers, are sunk in that limitless ocean. Brahman is both inside and outside of us. If through concentration we could keep ourselves saturated with the thought that this receptacle—the body, mind, and faculties—is nothing but a container, is it so difficult to believe we can realize Brahman? Constant thinking on the Ideal, concentrating on it while you are busy, brings realization more rapidly.

Here is a simple example. You are expecting a very dear person home after a long absence. He is arriving the day after tomorrow and you are busy from early morning till midnight making arrangements for his arrival. You have no time for any other thought. Both your body and mind are tremendously busy. Now, try to analyze the background of your consciousness. Can you remain separate from the thought of that beloved person? In the course of your intense activity, every action, every breath is controlled completely by that one thought. Even while cleaning your house you are thinking of your guest. When you are preparing the food, your hand might be peeling potatoes but your consciousness remains absorbed in the thought of that beloved person. That undercurrent of thought remains steady throughout all your thoughts and activity.

If you are willing to accept this little illustration, you should not hesitate to accept its larger meaning. The highest ideal must be thoroughly assimilated into our system as the basic principle of our living. Then, if need be, we can move safely about in this world of phenomena; but we will find, under all circumstances, that we remain attached to the basic principle of our being. And concentration is the means to the realization of the true nature of our Self, the Divinity.

Divinity is our consciousness in its pristine state. Whatever attributes we think of as pertaining to Brahman apply also to our consciousness. We think of Brahman as being omnipotent, immortal and so on. All of this is affirmed by our consciousness, which has these attributes as well. But when that Consciousness expresses itself through the instruments of our body and mind it appears to be limited; it seems to take upon itself the limitations of the instruments. If I raise this pencil in the air it is Consciousness that raises the pencil. It is Consciousness proper working through the instrumentality of this mechanism. But seeing this action, no one will think it is omnipotent. Why not? *Because we do not identify the Source with the action.* We do not recognize that power which acts through the instrumentality of the body and mind.

Consciousness proper, in its pristine state, without any superimpositions, separated from the qualities of the instruments, can be realized only by the process of meditation. We talk of meditation, but what is it? Meditation is the process of eliminating all the distorting conditions that interfere with that ever-present, pure Consciousness. In the process of meditation, first of all shut the doors of sensation. If you are able to do that, you find your consciousness in a different state. Think of a vast background of consciousness with five openings. If you close the openings (the senses) you will find your consciousness in a more concentrated form. But still there are subtle forms that limit it. There are impressions in your memory. Although your eyes do not now see them, you still think of things you saw previously. These impressions "stamp" the background of the Consciousness with form and colour. A printer of cloth takes his block and stamps a piece of white cloth with many colours and designs. Similarly, the mind is given form by the impressions made on it. If you eliminate the "stamps," the impressions of your consciousness, you at last get what you originally have. The process of realizing our real nature is the process of eliminating the limiting conditions. Then we recognize what we all the time were.

By stamping our self-consciousness with little object of possession and the desire to possess and to enjoy, we have become small like our desires. If you want to realize that pure state of Consciousness, which is Brahman, in its totality, then get rid of all those stamps. Yoga teaches us how to remain above that stamping of the consciousness. Yoga teaches you to refuse the little and gain the All. Anything you consider as your self, anything you attach yourself to only limits the real you. To give up, to renounce, means to refuse to stamp yourself with anything. Meditate upon the truth. Know that you are not action, not desire, not what you express. You are the substratum which expresses itself through all these functions. Always think of yourself as That which expresses itself in the expression. Do not become confused about that.

The limiting qualities, the upadhis, that stamp the consciousness make it *appear* to be what it is not. They are like cloaks that hide the reality in the internal as well as the external world. Now, we are only attached to these upadhis because we are concentrated on them. That is maya. Realization of the truth is accomplished by meditation, by eliminating the limiting conditions.

This consciousness of ours, which we sometimes call mind or intelligence, *is that Brahman*. But the absolute nature of Brahman has been hidden by layers and layers of impurities made up of ignorance. Gold is intrinsically pure and brilliant, but when it is mixed up with other substances it appears devoid of lustre. It looks like ordinary ore. This "substance" which we are handling every day, our consciousness, is a pure, precious metal, like gold. We have to eliminate the impurities from the gold.

In order to purify gold, the goldsmith follows a certain procedure. There are three steps in this process. The first is to remove the grossest layer of impurities that cling to the gold like a coating. To do this, the goldsmith puts the gold on the anvil and hammers and hammers it until these impurities are removed. Next, the gold must be rid of impurities which have adhered to it chemically. This requires a vigorous scrubbing and scouring. Even a strong chemical may be needed. Then there are more subtle impurities that can only be removed by putting the gold into fire. But after it comes out of this fire process, it is pure gold. The dross has been completely removed.

So it is with the removal of ignorance from the human con-sciousness. We are all going through these cleansing processes, knowingly or unknowingly. Although the student in spiritual life may be doing so knowingly, the process causes him a great deal of suffering. For is it not painful when we first learn that all that seems so real to us, and which we depend upon and cling to so desperately, is not real and lasting? Do we not suffer when our senses must be controlled and our desires curtailed? Is it not agonizing,sometimes, when our assertive ego has to be "hammered" again and again in order to be vanquished? Certainly it is painful.

In many religions, of course, suffering has been extolled, glorified. But mere suffering as suffering is no glory! Mere suffering will not do. If this were so, all the homeless and starving people in the world would be the holiest. When suffering becomes *consciously* purifying it will no more be thought of as suffering. Its burden will be much lighter. It is only by going through these processes which cause us suffering and pain for the time being that we can remove the ignorance ingrained in our consciousness. We must go through willingly, and with our eyes set determinedly on the goal.

Even at the last stage; however, when layer after layer of ignorance has been removed, our consciousness will still have some defect clinging to it. It will still retain an individual chara-cter, still be a solitary unity. A whirlwind might still overcome it and again throw it into a dust bin—because it is not yet the All. Unless and until it has become the All, become Brahman, it is not safe.

The state of being the All is called *nirvikalpa samadhi,* a state beyond all duality. That is the final goal of jnana yoga. Even if your consciousness, which is now full of doubt, grief, and so many other complaints, becomes a thousand times more pure, abounds in happiness and possesses great spiritual powers, that consciousness will still be the consciousness of an individual. So do not think that what it has attained will last forever. Of course, if your ideal is one of enjoyment you will be repelled by the thought of the nondualistic state anyway. You will say, as did one of the greatest of *bhaktas,* "I do not want to *be* sugar: I want to *eat* sugar!" The monist, on the other hand says, "All right, go ahead and eat sugar, but you will get a stomachache!" Freedom is attained only by "being sugar."

That final state of "being sugar" has been extolled by all the great spiritual teachers, men of the highest realization. And they have encouraged us not to stop until that goal of nirvikalpa samadhi is reached. We have to merge our individual self totally, into the ocean of *Sat-chid-ananda*—Existence, Knowledge and Bliss Absolute. There can be no compromise; that is the goal. When that is achieved, this container, our individual consciousness, will melt away; no more will there be any desire to return to individual consciousness. But will we lose anything? Certainly not. Brahman *includes* all; Brahman *is* the All, and by realizing Brahman we become the All. We become the universal Self, ever-existing, Knowledge itself, and Bliss inexpressible.

Total absorption, then, is the goal. Do not think that it is an easy task. First of all you have to convince yourself that there is no sense enjoyment that is lasting, either in this world or in other worlds. In the realm of phenomena, gross or subtle, there is bound to be limitation, which cuts at the very root of spiritual freedom. To make up one's mind to attain the state of nirvikalpa samadhi is to totally reject subject-object consciousness.

Those who have attained that state have never found adequate words to describe it, for we can only talk in terms of matter. Who can express the Inexpressible? But in poetic language, an attempt has been made. One poet wrote: "If ten thousand suns could shed their brilliance at one moment, they would appear weak before that Presence. If twenty million moons could focus their light at once, that would not compare with the radiance of that supreme Brahman." The simile of light has often been used in trying to describe Brahman.

This present consciousness of ours, no matter how it appears is that divine radiance beside which ten thousand suns and twenty million moons are pale and insignificant. Just think of that! So, let us begin with the process of removing our ignorance—by the "hammering, scrubing and firing" of our consciousness. Let us proceed with understanding, knowing that the goal will be reached when these initial processes have been gone through. Let us understand that every blow we may experience in life or in our spiritual endeavours is actually a blessing in disguise; for it helps us release self-consciousness from the clutches of the senses that the tie us down to subject-object consciousness. The process, no doubt, entails suffering. But it is not vainglorious, it is not self-torture.

It is, in actuality, self-analysis.

In jnana yoga, sravana, manana, and nididhyasana are the processes of purifying the "gold" of our consciousness; but they are mere "drops in the bucket" compared to nirvikalpa samadhi. Manana is reflection; it is superior to sravana, or hearing. The practice of manana is a hundred times superior to sravana. Nididhyasana, or meditation, is a hundred times superior to manana. But nirvikalpa samadhi, says Sankaracharya, is infinite in its results.

The disciplines prescribed in jnana yoga will purify the gold of our consciousness until it shines in its own pure, unalloyed splendour. This is nirvikalpa samadhi.

5

IN his contacts with the world, the follower of jnana yoga, so long as his consciousness retains the characteristics of an individual unit, always aspires to see the One behind the many. His ideal, if it can be expressed in very simple language, is to see the Truth—Brahman—everywhere, within and without. It is said that when he *does not see* anything but Brahman, *does not touch* anything but Brahman, *does not hear* anything but Brahman; in other words, when all his faculties have been completely saturated with the realization of the Reality, *That* shines out into everything, external as well as internal. The yogi has then attained consciousness of the unity behind all variety. He sees the variety, like all of us do, but he knows that Brahman alone is *real;* the universe (as a variety of forms) is unreal; and that his soul is nothing but Brahman.

The unity of the individual soul and Brahman, however, is not to be "attained." Unity is always unity. It must either exist at all times or not at all. It cannot be found sometime or somewhere. If I am not one and the same with the divine principle, Brahman, at this present moment, I cannot be so, say, two years from now. If I am not one with It in this present location, then though I travel throughout the universe, I shall never find a spot where I shall be.

If we admit this proposition at all—that finally we have to realize our unity with Brahman—we must admit that we are one with It now. No separation ever took place. It is only our false conception regarding our Self that has created this monstrous blunder that make us think we are separate from It. As a result of that ignorance we are compelled to think Brahman is far, far away from us. When the ignorance is removed, we find we have always been one with Brahman.

In explanation of this, I should like to make a general and very bold statement: unless and until the ideal for which we are striving is *already within us* we cannot beg, borrow or steal it anywhere in this world. For instance, do you think a person can understand the goodness or kindness of another unless he has such qualities developed within himself? I doubt it. You cannot see anything outside yourself which you do not carry within.

This applies negatively as well. If you cherish negative thoughts, you will find negativism everywhere. A thief thinks this a world of thieves. A selfish person ascribes selfish motives to everyone.

Therefore, unless you have the ideal of the realization of Brahman, you can never realize Brahman. If you expect the Reality to be somewhere in time and space, or in the hereafter, you will be disappointed. (I am, of course, speaking from a nondualistic point of view). If you want to find Brahman, you will have to discover it within your self. And when you do, and you make yourself saturated with that inward realization, you will know that whatever comes out of you is that Brahman which you perceive within. Then you will *know* that the individual soul, the universe, and Brahman are one and the same.

The highest goal of life is total absorption in that one, infinite Existence. So long as there are two, there will always be fear. Where there is duality and form there is time and space and, therefore, the possibility of transformation and change. So where are perfection and freedom in the presence of two? We are not considering this question from the standpoint of enjoyment; if we ask for that, we must remain in the dualistic state. But enjoyment will not always be sought. A time will come when you will be more concerned about perfection and freedom than mere enjoyment. One must transcend all desires, all consciousness of duality. Then the human soul will be realized as Brahman.

To perceive unity in variety has been the ideal of all wisdom. Even if we consider today's various scientific investigations, we find the endeavour is still to discover the One expressing itself in the forms of many. Let us direct our own investigations to the things that are in this room, for instance. If, finally, we find they are made of one substance, "X," we can say that we know "X," and that thus we know everything in this room. The craving for knowledge will be satisfied only when we have known the One out of which the many have come.

As a matter of fact, the One is always at the back of our consciousness. If our thoughts were only composed of various worldly impressions, without this "background" of Consciousness, our minds would always be in a state of turmoil. It would be a veritable tempest! So many vibrations would be entering our consciousness at the same time as to completely unbalance us. Fortunately, this is not the state of affairs. Though we might not be *aware* of the unity, it *is* that unity, nevertheless, that first registers on our consciousness; and it is on the basis of this unity that we form our conceptions of the variety. This is what prevents us from going mad! Analyze your daily contacts and you will find that there is a power which constantly merges variety into unity. For the moment, our consciousness may seem to be simply absorbing all the vibrations; there is upheaval and turmoil in our minds. But this settles down when, by the process of generalization, all is unified. In other words, all the "raw materials" of sound colour, smell, and so on are drawn within and merged into "X." As soon as they become "X," which forms the background of everything, we derive wisdom from our experiences. This process is going on unconsciously. But we can develop a special faculty for recognizing that common "X" first, and on the basis of that, recognizing all the variety.

We must know that the ultimate ideal of philosophy, of knowledge, is to find the unity in the variety in this universe. Make your own experiments, observe the variety, classify everything, but do that with the object of eventually being able to find out their common background. Identify a dog as a dog, a cat as a cat, and a horse as a horse. Examine them each as to their individual characteristics. Then go deeper and find something common to them all. Today you are interested in psychology, tomorrow biology, and the next day some other subject. Study each one scientifically, then go on, go deeper into these subjects; try to discover the one thread that runs through them all.

Take yourself as a subject for study. You may be a businessman, a writer, an artist, an office clerk—and a singer as well. In addition to any of these, you perhaps serve a role as a mother or father. Suppose that in the execution of your duties in any of these roles you lose your identity, that you fail to recognize your self—the thread of your being—in all your different relationships and vocations. You would be called a lunatic. Understand clearly that a continuous, unchanging principle forms the background of your self and your knowledge of things. If you once recognize the existence of that principle behind all the world's variety, subjectively and objectively, you will feel the need for cultivating the habit of always being consciously aware of it.

It is our attitude that brings home to us either the unity or the variety. If we look at the world from one angle it reveals the basic unity; from another angle it describes very sharply the outlines of each individual manifestation. I do not mean to say that you should lose all sight of the variety, but first recognize the fundamental principle that is common to all. We should be aware of the variety (in fact, we shall have to as long as we live), but we can do so in a harmonious and peaceful way. One has to be able to recognize the Substance expressing itself in variety. If you want to reduce all the books found in a bookcase into one, you must first begin with paper, ink, cloth, and so on. Though the subject-matter varies considerably, the books themselves consist of only a few materials. Of course, in the world of gross matter you cannot reach an ultimate conception of unity, though you can "narrow the field." To discover unity you must proceed deeper into the realm of the Spirit. If I want to recognize the unity behind you, or a group of human beings, and I consider only skin, eyes, hair, features, and so on, I might be able to generalize but I would not be able to narrow all of you to unity. However, if I go deeper and first realize the existence of a principle which manifests itself as my emotions, my intelligence, and my physical being, I would then find the same Spirit in everyone.

You must convince yourself that such a recognition is necessary. Ask yourself, "Do I want to recognize variety, or unity?" If you say only variety, I shall say, "All right, go ahead, but when you are sick and tired of it, come back to me. I shall point out where we agree, and following that thread of agreement we will finally reach unity."

The basic principle of existence, Brahman, is without any

diversity. It is because of that unity behind our consciousness that we are able to sense the universe in various ways. This universe of variety exists in the mind; by concentrating the mind on unity within, we shall gradually be able to eliminate variety from our minds and realize the One without diversity. But we have to make a beginning. First, gain an appreciation for that transcendental principle. Convince yourself that it is essential, absolutely necessary, for you to recognize it behind all your faculties. Without that conviction, no understanding of it will be possible. If this is just a matter-of-fact assertion, it will do little good. We must be in real earnest. We must become aware, more and more, of that Entity. That Entity is absolute and motionless; hence beyond action. It is beyond time, space, and causation. It is beyond the mind, but it is *reflected* in the purified ego. We become aware of that absolute Entity when we can detach our Self from the mind. We must dissolve the root of delusion, which is ignorance of our true Self. We have to get hold of that real "I," and we do so by eliminating, one by one, the consciousness of all those things we think it is. It is not the body, nor the senses, nor the faculties. It is not the mind. It is detached from everything we know, yet it is the background of everything we know. It is present always and everywhere but it eludes us, it escapes our grasp. It is what It is.

The fundamental and really the most important truth taught by jnana yoga is that the soul of man, the Self of man, is omnipotent, omnipresent and infinite in its nature. It is Sat-chid-ananda—absolute Existence, Knowledge and Bliss. Now, if we accept this proposition, what conception can we have regarding our Self or soul? What is its nature? First of all, we have to know that it is infinite, not bound by space or time. When you say "my soul!" you cannot think of it in terms of a little something which is implanted within your body. It is all-pervading, exists in all times, and occupies all space; so, in fact, you cannot say that your soul and the soul of a Christ or a Buddha (or that of the smallest insect, for that matter) are different. Does that shock you? But you simply cannot use the plural noun for the word, soul. There are no souls. There is only one, and in jnana yoga it is known as Brahman.

Brahman is the all-pervading, formless, Absolute Reality. It is not bound by the limitations of space, time, or causation. If you think of form you have to place it in space. It is then bound by the limitations of space; it is not all-pervading. As soon as you admit the limitation of space you admit the limitation of time; thus, form cannot be immortal. Then what is this formless, timeless reality which we may call the essence of existence?

Let us analyze this expression, "essence of existence." What do you think is the essence of existence? Make a long list of all the things that exist for you. Now try to name something that is the essence of them all. You may say there is none, or perhaps all of them taken together. You are mistaken. All these items are changing every moment. All the external objects you have listed, as well as your body, mind, and internal faculties, are changing every moment. Do you agree? But what we are seeking is That which does not change, for that which changes cannot be absolute. We are seeking the very essence of existence.

Now, who is the subject of all the objects on your list? Who are *you*? What constitutes *your* existence? Remember, you cannot say that it is the sum-total of these changing objects, for that would be a blunder in logic. If a thing is not contained in the individual items, the sum-total of them could not produce it. You have to admit that all of these items are held together by a "something" which is the ultimate subject of them, and which we may simply call Existence Absolute. All of these items are cognized by an Entity which does not change. There must be a changeless background to all change. It was St. Paul who said: "In Him we live, move, and have our being." By this is meant the transcendental essence of our existence. We cannot be, or move, or function unless that One supplies the background of power. This is not only so of human beings. but of every manifestation. Every manifestation floats on that infinite "ocean" of existence. It floats on it like a small bubble. It is always part of the ocean, never really different from its source. Or, again, we may say that it floats on the ocean like a piece of ice floats on water. And when the ice disappears, where does it go? It enters that very same water on which it floats. Where else could it go? Existence Absolute is that in which we "live, move , and have our being."

Because we give no consideration to anything except the qualities, the forms of the different manifestations that float on the ocean of existence, we do not recognize the background, that which is expressing itself through all the forms. The qualities, the forms, are limiting conditions. They "hide" the reality from us. Absolute Existence exists for its own sake and does not depend upon any qualities. Although it may be difficult at first, we can train ourselves to recognize that there is an Absolute Existence which is appearing in many forms, with qualities. Of course, it requires an exercise of our power of analysis to form a clear conception of this. But it can be done. Ask yourself. "Do I consider my existene to be my limbs, my head, my heart, my liver, or what?" Your existence is not associated with any of these, nor with their sum-total. There is, however, an Absolute Existence which is expressed by these appearances. Something has taken place on that background of existence. upon which all external existences are nothing but "arrangements"

It has also been stated that the essence of our soul, or Brahman, is Knowledge Absolute. It *is* knowledge itself, rather than having knowledge. We say, infinite Knowledge, absolute Knowledge. What do we mean? There is Knowledge proper (absolute Knowledge) and the knowledge of things. You have a background, a storehouse, of Knowledge and you are giving different forms to it. It is only the various expressions of Knowledge that differentiate it. If I say the word "water," what happens? Knowledge proper takes the form of water. Suppose that there is nothing in your mind for the time being but the remembrance of water. Has that exhausted your power to project knowledge? There are many Knowledge-forms bubbling up on the surface of your mind. If you were to ask me to recapitulate what I have seen on my recent trip around the world, Knowledge proper would immediately express itself in a variety of forms. Differentiated knowledge is only an expression of Knowledge proper. In fact, without the storehouse of Knowledge proper you could not project forms at all.

What do we know about that undifferentiated Knowledge proper? We know it is not knowledge like our knowledge of a tree, a bird, or a dog. It is *That* which expresses itself in and through our knowledge of things. And that power is flowing through every being, finding expression through everyone's knowledge. But that Knowledge is expressed only partially through individual consciousness. Let us take as an example an infinite ocean of heat which is manifested in a certain way here and another way there. Is it so hard to conceive of this? Although there exists a basic principle of heat *per se,* the temperature of heat is not the same every where. In a large blast furnace that principle of heat creates many degrees of temperature; in a refrigerator it manifests in a different way. Let us go back to our proposition: Brahman, or the Reality, is infinite Knowledge which manifests itself through the different media of body, mind, and consciousness. Suppose you know so much, someone else a little more, and so on. That knowledge is God, but it is not all of God. God, the Reality, is infinite, Knowledge is infinite. Knowledge is manifesting itself according to the capacity of the containers. Your knowledge is God, your existence is God; only it is expressed partially, according to the capacity of your individual container Can you conceive of that infinite substratum, irrespective of your or my container? Is it possible? We know that the light of the sun is reflected onto many different things. We know the reflections are of the same sun, though they appear very differently. We also know that all the various colours are but different graduations of one light. It is not difficult to conceive of the background of the different manifestations of light, is it? Can we not conceive of the background of all the knowledge that is expressed through different manifestations, or containers, bodies and minds? Consider your knowledge as a ray of God, the reality, and that God, the background and source of all your knowledge, as omnipotent, omnipresent, and unlimited. Knowledge proper is Brahman, the essence of your being.

There is another descriptive aspect of Brahman which we have not touched on: that Brahman is infinite Bliss. Bliss is very difficult to define. In fact, it can only be described in negative terms. It is that condition of your consciousness in which you have no want of any kind, no conflict, no worry or suffering, no limitation of any sort to your happiness and peace. The condition that we all experience, and that may be considered as the nearest to Bliss, is the state of deep, dreamless sleep. The analogy of deep sleep to Bliss signifies that the way to attain infinite Bliss, which is the essence of our existence, is to put our faculties to sleep, our senses, mental functions, memory—all. Put them to sleep. The result will be Bliss. When you awake from the state of deep sleep you say, "Oh, how peacefully I slept! No nightmares, no dreams. My headache disappeared. I forgot my worries, my pains and troubles." Everything is denied, eliminated. Bliss is that state in which there is absence of limitation of any kind. It is that which remains when we have eliminated all limiting conditions. A little bit of that Bliss comes out through the senses. We call it happiness. When the senses contact objects which bring pleasurable sensations, although they do not last, although they may be only momentary, they create adulterated forms of that Bliss which we have within us. We distort that Bliss when we bring it down into the realm to phenomena. It is Bliss distored, Bliss disfigured. I have seen a·dog chewing on a rubber toy, an artificial bone. The dog takes it and goes to a secluded corner and lies down and starts to chew on the "bone". He chews and chews until it is covered with his saliva, and perhaps, his gums bleed, too. Only then it seems, does the bone taste good to him, for he is quite content to lie in the corner and chew on it. It is his own saliva he is licking from the bone, yet that gives him happiness. In a similar way, it is our own Bliss that is issuing through our senses and we are enjoying it.

We should try to understand that there is the *Thing* expressed, and there are its expressions, its attributes. The Absolute contains the potentiality of all qualities, but the trouble is that the attributes, the qualities, have become the reality to us. If we can gain a conception of the *Thing* which is being expressed, then we will know that all life is an expression of Absolute Existences, all knowledge a ray of Absolute Knowledge, and all happiness (in fact, all sensations) are expressions of that Absolute Bliss, although distorted and sometimes disfigured by the qualities. Then and then alone will we know that our real nature is Sat-chid-ananda.

Let us go back to our proposition: Brahman pervades all space, exists in all time. It is omnipotent, omniscient, limitless and indescribable. It is my soul, my essence. My existence, my knowledge, depends upon That; my bliss, my happiness, is a manifestation of that infinite Bliss which is my essence.

Suppose there is an infinite expanse of water, a limitless ocean. In it are immersed bottles of various shapes, forms, and colours, Like those bottles, we individuals are immersed in the infinite ocean of Brahman that fills up every container, every one of us, like the water filling the bottles immersed in it. The differences are in the containers, not in the contained substance. Brahman is the one Substance which pervades everything. It is the basic principle, the background, of our knowledge, our bliss, and our very existence. If we think about our existence we can only think of That. If we think of knowledge, we can only think of that

Knowledge which is God, or Brahman, and if we feel any happiness, or bliss, it is that Bliss which is God, the essence of our existence. Well, that is the situation. We are all "containers" of different shapes and forms, like the bottles in our simile. And we are all moving about in the infinite "ocean" of Brahman. Why have we come to be in these forms? I cannot answer that. We call it maya but, as Swami Vivekananda said, that is only a "statement of fact," not an explanation. I must build my conclusion on the fact that I find it like this. I can only go forward, not backward.

The practical question would be, aside from all philosophical considerations; what can be done with these containers? In other words, what is your aim and object? Every container has taken on an individuality and each one is moving in that Substance. Why? Just because it wants to. The individual container wants to move about, because it wants to retain its individuality. That is the only explanation. Suppose, as it is moving as a small unit and experiencing different things, it has a desire to become like some bigger container it sees. It looks at it longingly and thinks: "I would like to be like *that!*" Then, gradually, urged on by that desire, it evolves into that which it wanted to be. It goes on and on in such a manner, evolving towards a more and more perfect container. Now, when such a container reaches a certain point in its evolution, what happens to it? What attitude does it develop towards the Substance within, towards the "ocean" in which it moves? It says, "I do not want to retain the consciousness of being separate, of being a container, any more. *I want to be one with the ocean.* The ocean has fullness of Existence, Knowledge, and Bliss. By experiencing all these different forms of containership, I was only partially experiencing what I actually desired." No matter what the size or quality of the container may be, it is only a "drop in the ocean." A time comes when one feels like that, when one feels the oppressive nature of all containers, when one decides one wants to be through with all limitations.

Has this given you a hint as to what is known as reincarnation? The individual goes on evolving and evolving as long as the desire for individuality remains. But are we to go on in this way forever? Is there no release from it? When you understand the theory of reincarnation, then you want to trample it underfoot. If you once really understand that the "ocean of Brahman" is the basic reality of your being, that you *are* the ocean, you will be able to give up this clinging to individuality. If you once get even a glimpse of That with which you are filled, you will know that there is no need to preserve your container, your individuality. The highest truth is that all containers are a bondage and a prison. But until you reach that stage of understanding, use your container (body, mind and faculties) wisely. It will help you. Give it proper rest, nourishment, and discipline. It will help you and lead you on. But know that this is not the highest truth, not the full truth. You are caught in a maze of containers. Get out of it as soon as possible!

People often say that the idea of reincarnation gives them a good deal of consolation; it makes them happy to know that death is only a change of bodies. But I do not think it is a consolation at all. That a slave is again to be born as a slave—is that any consolation? Most people shudder at the thought of giving up their individuality. They cling to it with all their might because they have identified themselves with it. They have no idea of the Substance within them. What if it were established that when death came the container would break and all be over? I for one would say, "fine!" But reincarnating again, coming again and again into this bondage, remaining separate—when are we going to be through with it all? When there will be no more container. Death is only the changing of the form of the container, changing the "bottle" from round to square, to oblong and on and on. Death does not dispose of the container, of the tendency to take on another container. It just changes the container to another shape. The release from this bondage can only come from the realization that you *are* the fullness of Existence, Knowledge, and Bliss. Anything short of that is a bondage.

Now, how do we assimilate and understand this? We have to discriminate constantly between the "container" and the "contained." We have to become more and more aware that all containers are filled with one and the same Substance. And we have to pay more attention to the contained than to the container. We have to think: *here,* the contained Substance is appearing in this form; *there,* that container is filled with the same Substance. Do this repeatedly, intensely, and sincerely for six months and you will see what difference it will make in your outlook. Your consciousness will expand; limited boundaries of thinking will begin to disappear, and you will live in the light of a new understanding. Then with this new understanding, read the spiritual teachings of all the great Masters. You will find much more light in them.

This truth, reached by the method of jnana yoga, by discrimination, is the last word in spirituality. You may attempt to realize the Truth by some other process, some other method, but this is the final expression: you must know Brahman, *be* Brahman, right now, in this present life. Sankaracharya said in his "half a verse" that the jiva (individual soul) is nothing but Brahman. This has to be realized in this very life, and a jnani will not stop short of it.

The follower of jnana yoga is convinced that knowing the Truth, realizing his own self as Brahman, is the goal of life. But is he to know this as he knows any object? You say, "I perceive—I know—this flower." What has happened? Like a searchlight, you projected a sort of light of understanding through your senses; with the help of that light, by a process of knowing within you, the flower was comprehended. You were the knower and the flower was the known. You were the subject and the flower was the object. Now, are we to know Brahman as we know this flower? Would you be satisfied if you knew Brahman, or the Truth, as you know an object? You would not, and I will tell you why. Any object that you know occupies space, exists in time, and is influenced by the law of causation. It is, therefore, subject to change. Any object that you can know objectively has limitations; hence, it cannot have absolute existence. It cannot be perfect. How, then, can it be the final truth? No object can be the ideal we are seeking. We have to know the Subject of all objects.

By searching into objects, or the knowledge of objects, no solution to the problem can be found. *You must turn within.* At first we try to solve the problem by searching into objects and possessing them. We search in the external world, in the objects of perception. Then, after a long time, we discover that this is not the way. There is always the duality of seeker and sought of subject and object. We find we cannot go beyond this duality.

Then you turn within. Of course, you still have the consciousness of being a seeker, of seeking to comprehend the inner light of understanding. The duality remains. But you begin to realize that whatever object you perceive is revealed according to your understanding, to the light you shed upon it. No object in this world, no matter what it is, reveals itself as it is. Again, it appears to you in the light of understanding you shed upon it. Now, in continuing your search, you want to know what that is. (This is a most difficult time.) You are analyzing your own understanding. But you will not be able to know what that is until the seeker merges himself into the sought, or *vice versa*. The seeker and the sought have to be merged into one, and when that happens, out flashes the truth. Can you call such a state knowledge? It is not knowledge, as we understand it, because knowledge presupposes a subject and object. Where there is no object, what is there to be known? It simply *is*. That is all that can be said of it. The one who was seeking into everything, first in the external and then in the internal world, is revealed *as the thing sought*. You are seeking something; all of a sudden the understanding flashes within you that *you* are the thing sought. There language fails. No expression is possible in that state. That is revelation, or samadhi. When you realize the self, or the seeker, as the object sought you discover the highest culmination of Existence, Knowledge and Bliss—Sat-chid-ananda. You become That. It is not that you know God, or Brahman, the Reality; I say you become It.

Now, what is the difference between the two states of consciousness, when you had the consciousness of being a seeker, and after your real Self is realized? What is the difference between sense knowledge and revelation? When you are going through the analysis process, you say to yourself: "I am seeking; I feel I have a consciousness, a mind, body, and senses. I consider myself imperfect. I am seeking perfection."

Before the truth is realized, you have superimposed many ideas upon that Reality. These ideas are false. Make any statement about yourself. You will find that you are either affirming or denying qualities to yourself. You may say, "I am mortal, imperfect, and weak." Or, "I am strong and happy." Both these affirmations and denials are superimpositions. You falsely ascribe such qualities to your self, without knowing its real nature. And such is the power of the superimpositions that the results manifest themselves in you, even though these things never touch the real you! (The classical example of superimposition is the rope and the snake simile mentioned earlier.) Here, in the case of our self-consciousness, all statements that we make are nothing but superimpositions. When the superimposed qualities are eliminated from the "I", then the "I" reveals itself as the divine reality.

Is it possible for us, by exercising our power of reasoning, to comprehend that the divine principle is our own self? Is it possible for us to know that it is that principle which is expressing itself in and through all our feelings, thoughts, and actions? It is true that it cannot be an object of the mind, the mind cannot picture it. But as we proceed, reasoning with discrimination, we find that this truth unfolds itself in our understanding. We begin to feel that there is a universal power which is expressing itself in forms, which animates forms, and speaks and acts through them. But, you may ask, what about all the defects we see? Are they divine expressions? If we find defects in any expression they should be ascribed to the machinery through which the divine force is expressing itself. We explain the defects in the transmission of electrical energy in terms of the machinery through which it is transmitted, or expressed. We do not say the energy is defective. Likewise, we should attribute all differences and defects to the machinery, or the transmitter (body and mind)—not to the Substance which flows through it.

You may think that since the body and mind are only "machinery," we can neglect them altogether. That is not so. In fact, there is even scope for improving this machinery just as we improve common machines. But, in the long run, what would be the outcome of your attempts to improve this machinery? Perhaps you could extend its capabilities; still it would not be perfect. Suppose you want to bring home the ocean. The first day you go with a pint bottle, but you find it is too small. So you go on increasing the size of the container to a quart and to a gallon. But if you want the ocean, you must have the ocean as your container. In other words, you cannot bring it home. You have to go to the ocean. Improve and develop the machinery of your body, mind, senses and other faculties as much as you want, but know that you can never develop a machinery that will be powerful enough to express completely the Spirit. You will have to throw away all machinery. The machinery is all right and serves its purpose, but we must learn to pay more attention to the inner Substance. If we go on denying That, here within, and in the objects we contact, I call it ignorance, worldliness, materialism, and death. Whereas, if we admit the existene of a power, a Divinity, which is present in the subject as well as the object, and if we recognize, also, the limited conditions for what they are, as machinery through which that power expresses itself, I call that spirituality. That is knowledge.

As you proceed in this manner you will find a calmness in the depth of your being you did not feel before. The importance of external circumstances and appearances will become minimized. By directing our consciousness towards the Source within we are able to remain peaceful and calm under all the trying circumstances we meet in life. In the Gita it is said that one who attains that state of steady understanding is like the ocean. If you pour millions of gallons of water into the ocean it will make no differene to it. The ocean is a reservoir, whose substance is being disposed of in various ways and, at the same time, is rushing into the ocean from so many different sources. But the ocean always looks just the same. Here, in the "ocean" of our consciousness, comes honour, dishonour, wealth, poverty; 'sometimes sickness, sometimes health; youth, and old age. Now, think of our little reservoir. What a difference even if one drop is added or subtracted! If something we possess is taken away from us, we lose our poise. We become completely upset. Then again, if one grain is added to us, if sudden success and praise come to us, we are equally disconcerted. From the view point of our tranquillity, the gaining of twenty thousand grains or the loss of twenty thousand grains is the same. But a person who has realized the truth, even intellectually, acts in an even manner in every situation.

One of the first signs of a person's advancement towards truth is his tranquillity under all circumstances. Even if inner poise leaves him once in a while, it does not take him long to regain it. Latu Maharaj [Swami Adbhutananda] used to tell us that anger—or lack of tranquillity—in a man of spiritual understanding is like writing on water. One second it exists; the next it disappears. Such a person can direct himself to the Source of his being and quickly regain his equanimity. It might be difficult for us to do this in the beginning, but if we keep the ideal before us, we will never feel ourselves separate from the divine Source;

we can always direct our consciousness to it. The secret is to be convinced, without any doubt, that *the divine Substance exists, and that we can draw from It.*

It is said that for a man of such steadiness of understanding, for such a knower of truth, the world does not exist. It means that he has discovered something behind this world of the senses which is more real than that which appears on the surface of it. So he moves in his own world. And where did he get that world? He developed a " light " of spiritual understanding that penetrates into the Reality and he always accepts the superimposed qualities, *as* superimposed qualities, not as the Reality. Sometimes you may almost get that clear vision. For intsance, when you look upon a vast crowd of people, you can almost feel there is but one substance moving in them, one reality peeping out from the various forms, expressing itself in all that variety. If that inner vision is once experienced, even momentarily, the remembrance is so strong it will never leave you. Did you ever look at a small child playing? Try to concentrate on understanding the child. Pay no attention to what he looks like, forget the environment. Just think of his mind, and that through it *something* is expressing itself. If you can intensify your concentration, the child will almost vanish, and you will find Brahman expressing Itself through the child. You will have a glimpse of Brahman.

In India they have kite-flying contests. The kites are made of coloured papers, with many different and sometimes beautiful designs. The kite string is covered with a resin-like solution containing ground glass, in order to cut the string of your opponent's kite. Now, if your kite string is cut, you do not go after the kite. You let it go. But little boys love to catch a kite that has been cut off. I was once sitting in a solitary place. I saw a little boy gazing up at a beautiful kite sailing in the sky. How he was praying that the kite would get cut away! And it did. The kite came slowly down, and the little boy ran after it. Though it came down quite low, the string remained too high for his reach. He came to the edge of a river, stood on his tiptoes, stretched his arms out as much as he could, but still could not reach the string. Just at that point something beautiful happened. A boatman came along and he said to the little boy, " Jump in !" The little boy eagerly obeyed, and the boatman rowed his boat after the kite, which was gradually coming lower and lower. Finally, the little boy caught hold of the string.

I was quietly watching all this ; then something happened to me. I could see nothing but bliss in that boy. I saw bliss flashing out of the boy when he caught the kite string. The only thought in the mind of the little boy had been, "If *only* I could reach the kite string!" And when at last he caught hold of it, all his desires, agitations, fears, anxieties, apprehensions—all the superimpositions —were gone. When these ceased to occupy his consciousness, then the Bliss of Brahman was projected. For the moment that boy was all Brahman. For me, externals were nearly completely eliminated, leaving only the internal bliss. It is a matter of the blotting out the externals. If you can do that, you gain a different outlook. You do not give so much importance to externals; and this outlook keeps you in constant touch with the Reality. You do not move in the external world in the same way any more.

If the scriptures, then, say that a knower of truth walks away from phenomena, from ignorance, what can you understand from this? How do you interpret it? Here is the apartment of ignorance; there the apartment of knowledge. He simply does not enter the room of ignorance any more. It is often said that he does not enter into the life of activity any more; but do not take this literally. It means that he lives in the constant awareness of the Reality. He is merged in Brahman. Where is there any activity in That? He knows that activity is only in the instruments. In that context, cessation of activity means that he has discovered the inner Reality behind all moving appearances.

We must become thoroughly convinced about the existence of Brahman within us and know it is That which is expressing itself through our activities and functions. Let such understanding unfold more and more. Let your consciousness be absorbed by that Consciousness, and whatever is expressed by you will be nothing but the radiation of divine power. Whatever you contact in the external world will be that same Brahman which is within you.

Now, if we take it for granted that each one of us is working for the attainment of spiritual illumination, the question arises : "What is our conception of such illumination?" It is often described as the attainment of spiritual light. When your understanding is unfolding, you feel it very much like light. Think of a light that is kindled within you, and, think of it as revealing the different phases of your being. It reveals the darkest corners of your self to you. It lays bare the workings of the inner man. We can describe that light as the absence of darkness. Darkness generates fear and creates many misconceptions ; it causes chaos and confusion in our minds. Darkness is the greatest symbol of ignorance. Spiritual light is the absence of all this. We may call it knowledge, true knowledge.

That inner light also shows you what the motive should be that impels your thoughts, feelings, and actions. In the final analysis, there can be only one motive behind all action and that is to let that divine light within shine out without obstruction. Let us suppose we have a light there. We cover it with all sorts of shades. The light is now obstructed; it will not shine out. It will seem almost nonexistent. Similarly, whatever ideas, whatever motives, we may superimpose on that inner spiritual light, that one true motive to action, will be in error and rob it of its power of manifestation.

A person of spiritual illumination has the true motive behind all actions and expressions. Every action, every feeling and thought of his, is motivated by that vitalizing light within. He feels its presence and then follows it without causing any obstruction to its expression. What is the main obstacle that obstructs that true spiritual motive? A distorted self-consciousness. The ego-consciousness distorts and limits the expresssion of the light within. But, by practice, you can keep your self-consciousness comparatively clear of such distortions and, at the same time, be efficient and wise and manifest that light in any field of endeavour. It requires constant vigilance and practice in order to clear the self-consciousness of excessive egoism.

Have you ever observed a small child, say a child of five, when he is making a castle of sand on the beach? I have watched this on the beach at Lake Michigan. He is busy doing something. And what is the condition of his self-consciousness? He is just *doing*. He is not thinking of how his work will be accepted, if his name will appear in the newspapers tomorrow, or if he will be praised for it. He is just doing. At that moment he is a great, unattached worker. Nothing is distorting that divine light within him. This is an example of undistorted self-consciousness. In it there is great power, because it is free from the limiting motive of ego-consciousness.

One of the first signs of illumination is freedom from self-consciousness. No matter what he does, such a person can only emit light and power through the expression of his faculties. The channels through which the light passes are all clear and clean, because they are free from self-consciousness. No darkness can come out of him any more. Whatever he does can only please and do good, can only be of benefit to all. He has become goodness, and for that reason whatever comes out of his " container" is nothing but goodness.

Imagine that you are made of glass, and that a light is shining within you, revealing all the workings of your inner being. Now, that light within you, the man of glass, also emits a kind of glow outside. It creates a circle of light all around you. It shines out wherever you go, and anything coming within the circumference of that light attains a special character and beauty, because of the light you are carrying within you. Spiritual light shines both in the subjective and the objective fields of life. Illumination is something like that. It reveals everything within, and sheds its light and power all around.

Many people ask: what actually happens when one becomes spiritually illumined? It is said that such a person enters into a state of consciousness called ecstasy. Is it possible to give any description of that state? It can only be expressed vaguely. If we can imagine the highest form of happiness we have ever experienced, and then imagine it multiplied a thousandfold and extended for the longest period conceivable, that might give us some idea of spiritual ecstasy, or the attainment of freedom. Jnana yoga emphasizes that aspect of realization—the attaiment of freedom.

What idea do we usually have about ecstasy? We think of something happening that has stirred up some of our inner faculties, the result being that a change has taken place within us, and we feel excessively happy. This is true and not true. No doubt, something has happened that has made us realize such a state of happiness. Suppose you are told that a very dear friend is dead. Then, after a long, long time he suddenly stands in front of you—alive! What is your reaction? You are dumfounded. Though you are extremely happy, even ecstatic, you cannot express yourself. None of your faculties work. Then the low tide of your ecstasy follows, and you embrace your friend and talk to him, almost incoherently at first, with tears of joy in your eyes.

But at the height of ecstasy no communication, no outburst of expression, is possible; ecstasy is such that it robs you of everything else. It occupies the whole of your being. In the state of spiritual ecstasy, or union of the self with the Self, all your functions and faculties cease. The Self stands apart, as it were, in its own intrinsically unagitated state. You are then in your primordial, natural condition of existence.

So, briefly, we may say that ecstasy is a state of being where there is the absence of all agitating, disturbing, limiting conditions. And it is not borrowed, it is not generated. It is your *real* nature. Some form of stimulation may be involved but it does not produce that state. Your real Self is in a state of nonagitation; for that reason we call it blissful. The realization of ecstasy is nothing but the capability of entering that natural, unagitated, blissful state of the real Self at will. According to jnana yoga, when you eliminate the whole universe from your consciousness, the result is a state of divine ecstasy.

The student following the method of jnana yoga is taught the art of cutting away the gross external world from the Self. If you shut your senses the external world will be partially eliminated. But it stil exists in your memory. By shutting the external "doors" you have gone in one step; but another wall stands in front of you. It is the wall of thoughts and memories. You have to apply a different technique to pull down this wall. Next you find there is the wall of self-consciousness, the feeling of "I am" Although your self-consciousness has expanded, having been freed from the limiting conditions of the senses and other faculties, yet it still prevents your entering the state of final ecstasy. The "I am" consciousness still remains. When, at last, this consciousness, the "I", vanishes, you merge into the Ocean of Reality. That is bliss of ecstasy. You are full of bliss, complete in knowledge, and in existence, limitless. You are free.

The words of those who have attained that state of final freedom communicate the strongest conviction to our hearts. Their statements are not like those of other men over which we often reason and argue to be convinced of their truth. In this connection, I should like to point out the difference between two sorts of statements: argumentative statements, and statements made by the force of realization. When a teacher makes an argumentative statement he stimulates the power of reasoning in his listeners. But when a teacher makes a statement based on the highest spiritual realization he *convinces the mind* of the hearer without reasoning or argument. In Sanskrit there is an expression, *siddhanta vakyam*, meaning, the successful, the final climax, of speech or utterance, a statement which had attained the climax of success. Such a statement can only be made by the power of spiritual realization, and it can only come from a living source. If Sri Ramakrishna tells you you are Brahman, what a difference than if I say so! His is, without doubt, a *siddhanta* expression.

Do not think that a siddhanta statement is just something you accept through reverence, awe, or fear. What you accept in that way does not sink very deep within you. You may be overpowered by a great personality, but when you go home you find that the statements he made are creating within you strong objections. Suppose you go to a great scholar and hear from him a profound statement. You feel sure it must be true and you accept it; but, later, in reconsidering it, various arguments and bubbles of doubts arise in your mind. Know that that was not a siddhanta statement. The distinguishing feature, the criterion, of a siddhanta expression is that it removes you from the region of doubt. You may not be able to fully realize the truth of the statement immediately, but doubt will vanish. And it comes to you in that way only from a living source. I speak from my own experience, for I have known living sources of spiritual power.

As we all cannot have these experiences, we have to be stimulated by argument and reasoning. But blessed is the man who has the opportunity of contacting, even through literature, siddhanta expressions that remove doubt and lift one into a new region of understanding. That is why the reading of books that contain siddhanta statements is so important in spiritual life.

According to the scriptures, spiritual illumination, or the state of realization, produces three basic effects in the aspirant. First, it is said that *all the " knots " of the heart, of the understanding, are severed.* The word, knots, is very apt. Did you ever try to untie the knots of a parcel ? Then you know how tightly bound they are, and how difficult it is to untie them. There are many "knots" in our consciousness. They have made their home in the ego-consciousness. In the " I am" consciousness are concealed all entanglements. But the fundamental knot is mistaking the unreal for the real. If we can loosen that one knot all others will be loosened of themselve. The Sanskrit word *granthi* means knot. *Chit-jada-granthi* means the tie, or the knot, that fastens the *chit* [intelligence] with *jada* [matter]. The thing that ties up reality with appearances creates all our confusion and it becomes difficult for us to distinguish between them. But, having removed that fundamental knot, other knots will be removed as a matter of course. How do we untie that knot? Suppose you want to get rid of a rope that is tangled up in knots. What will you do ? Apply a little spask of fire at one end of the rope and it will soon be burnt to nothing. Even if scme ash remains, even if the rope retains its form, just blow gentl and it will disappear. The secret is to put a spark of fire at one end of the rope, a spark from the fire of discrimination. Without discrimination it is not possible for us to untie the knots in our consciousness.

Second, it is said that *all doubts are removed.* doubts appear as the result of our not knowing the truth. When we have once known the truth there is no more doubt. Knowledge flows uninterruptedly.

Third, the scriptures say that *all karma dies out.* That means that you do not forge any new chains to bind you. We usually act according to the law of causation. We know that the chain of causation controls a good part of our lives. But when you realize the highest truth, that chain is broken because you no longer act from the sense of ego. Your actions as a free agent cannot bind you and create any further karma. When you know you are absolutely free, your intrinsic nature is beyond doing or not doing. The popular definition of freedom in Sanskrit is "to be able to do or not to do, as one wishes." When you are at liberty to do or not to do a thing, you are free.

A person of such spiritual illumination has realized his self as the Self of all. He has complete realization of the essence, *chit,* that of which knowledge is composed that which comprises the subject and the object. His ego-consciousness has vanished. He is established in Brahman. He is free, full of bliss, complete, full. And fullness knows no agitation.

The final state of being, the attainment of absolute perfection, is what is meant, in this philosophy , by the term "freedom." What would you do if you wanted to be free? You might say, "Well, in the first place, I should try to control everything. Then nothing can interfere with me." But I should reply, "That is like a master's rule over his slave. Such control is not freedom." Science is trying to control the forces of external nature to utilize them for man's benefit. But is science thereby leading us towards freedom? Or are we letting those forces merely use us, making us more and more helpless ?

The burden of the song of civilization has always been control and more control, control of power, of money, of resources and commodities, control of one group by another, and so on. The more "things" a man has under his control, the more he fools himself that he is free. While material science has developed through the attempt to control external nature, another science, the science of the spirit, has been progressing with absolute freedom as its goal. Even if we could be established in freedom from all external nature, we would still have to face our internal nature. Freedom from both is the highest goal of man.

The experience of nirvikalpa samadhi, the highest goal of man according to jnana yoga, cannot be expressed in human language. It has never been successfully described by any seer. Sri Ramakrishna used to say that Brahman is the only entity or thing that has not been defiled by word of mouth. Everything else can be talked about; but not Brahman. Things can be described in terms of quality, dimension, and so on, ; but in that state the consciousness of subject and object is united and all relative consciousness left behind. There is no "I" or "you" ; there is no seer or object seen. Everything is One, and that Oneness cannot be described. Although Sri Ramakrishna made many attempts to describe that state as he was experiencing it, his words vanished in the course of the description. He could go only so far; then the consciousness of the relative world merged in absolute Consciousness, and speech left him. There was no individual left to describe that state, nor anyone to whom to describe it. In that state of unity all modifications of consciousness are absent. Thus unity cannot be described.

Among those who aspire to the highest spiritual realization, only those of a certain type, perfect from birth [called Iswarakotis], can experience the fullness of nirvikalpa samadhi and return to ordinary consciousness. When other aspirants, classed as jivakotis, enter into that state of nonduality they never return to relative consciousness. What this means is that when a drop of water falls into the ocean, it does not come out to take the form of a drop again. It becomes one with the ocean. When that state is reached by a jivakoti his body drops off like a dry leaf. But shall we use the ordinary expression and say that he dies? No, he does not die. His real Self becomes separated from the material frame and enters the Source from which it came. Actually, the superimposition of identity, his identification with the frame, vanishes, leaving the Self *as it always was*—the indivisible Brahman.

Sri Ramakrishna gave a very beautiful illustration of what happens to one who attains nirvikalpa samadhi. A little salt doll wanted to measure the depth of the ocean. It went down to the ocean and stepped into the water. But as soon as it did so, what happened? It dissolved, it became one with the ocean. There was no one to measure it or to come back! That describes what happens to a jivakoti who reaches the highest state of samadhi. But such is the great power of the Iswarkotis that, although they can "dissolve in the ocean" and become one with Brahman, they can also come back again and assume their individual forms.

There are two opinions in Hindu philosophy regarding the state of consciousness in which those who have attained liberation reside before merging completely into nirvikalpa samadhi. Sri Ramakrishna described the state as that of a *jivanmukta*, one who is free while living in the body, free while apparently acting like one who is bound. He gave the simile of a sword of steel which, after touhng the Philosopher's Stone, is turned into gold. It retains the shape and form of a steel sword, but it cannot injure anyone. A jivanmukta has touched the Philosopher's Stone of absolute Consciousness. His entire being has been transformed. He still retains the size and form of a human body, but there is no bondage or imperfection in him. His lower self does not really exist, for he always identifies himself with the higher Self. Of course, he might feel hunger and thirst; he might feel the need of sleep and rest. But this does not mean that his consciousness is identified with the body. He treats the body, mind, and emotions as so many instruments. He known that his real Self is always detached from them. He acts only for the benefit of others. His actions are without self-interest; they are for the good of all.

Another opinion holds that there remains a slight touch of imperfection in the jivanmukta until he has transcended the body and mind completely through the continuous experience of unitary existence. However, such controversial matters need not engage

our attention at the present time. In this life we may not be able
to enjoy even a fraction of that highest samadhi, but in our attempt
to reach it let us endeavour to manifest in our character a few
traits of perfection. In time, we shall reach the goal.

The jivanmuktas remain in the relative world after realization in order to teach others. A little story illustrates the difference
between those who remain in the world and those who become
absorbed in Brahman. Two men were walking in a forest when
they came upon a walled enclosure which seemed to be a garden.
Music and other joyous sounds were heard coming from the garden.
It drew them irresistibly towards it. One of the men constructed
a ladder and climbed to the top of the high wall. He looked into
the enclosure and shouted for joy. Without a comment he threw
up his arms in ecstasy and jumped into the garden. The second
man also climbed to the top of the high wall. He saw the same
scene, but restrained himself, and after coming down the ladder
he called those who were nearby, and helped them to reach the
top of the wall.

This latter person is the teacher type. But do not think that
because of his concern for others, he is greater than the man who
jumped into the garden. By his attainment of complete freedom
from the body and mind, from all forms of maifestation, he greatly
influences those who aspire to reach that state of realization. Both
types are equally great; they are simply different.

Sometimes people say, "What good are those men who become
immersed in samadhi and do not remain to teach others ? Are
they not very selfish?" My reply is : "Can you and I judge?"
A shoemaker judges everything by his own standard. A potato
merchant was once asked if he wanted to buy a diamond, and he
said, "Yes." The other man then asked, "How much will you
give me for it?" "Ten pounds of potatoes," replied the merchant.
It is like that. We compute the worth of such holy men according
to our own standards. We dealers in potatoes want to appraise
the value of those of the highest spiritual realization in terms of
potatoes.

After Swami Vivekananda had attained the nirvikalpa state
as a young man, he wanted to remain in that state. But Sri Ramakrishna told him that he had many things yet to do. "Why be so
anxious to remain absorbed in that state?" he said. "Know
that it is yours. But I shall keep it locked up, like a treasure in

a box. When you have finished the work you have come here to do, I shall give you the key, then you can have your treasure."

That happened to two giant personalities. What about us pigmies? We must aim at the nirvakalpa state. We must endeavour to transcend every bit of manifestation. Then, if there is any reason why we should not become absorbed in Brahman, if there is anything we are to do in this world, we will be made to do it. If we have the attitude of wanting to help humanity, from the viewpoint of jnana yoga it is nothing but an excuse, an " alibi", for remaining in the world. It is just feeding the ego, nothing but that.

Everything will go on just the same if you or I do not contribute anything to this world. In fact, only those who are completely unattached to the world can render any service to it. Others only grind their own axes. He who can make up his mind that he wants nothing but absolute freedom will attain it. The guru or God will come with the "key" and open the "treasure box" for him. If any humanitarian work, or service to God or man, is to be done by him, it will be collected like taxes. Even if he is not eager to pay, the taxes will be collected all the same! If you have anything to do in the world after realization, you will be made to do it. You need not anticipate that. But if you cherish the desire of returning to this world after realizing the highest samadhi, I would have to ask you, "What do you really want? The highest realization, or the world?" If you cherish any desire you will never be able to attain realization

An aspirant must be completely desireless—of either heaven, hell, or any other place. He must have no wish to remain or to go anywhere. We have to be able to look at the sun without protective glasses. For us, the only ideal, the only goal, should be total absorption in the final state of nirvikalpa samadhi, into the absolute truth, Brahman. Nothing short of that must be sought. Everything else is maya.

II

RAJA YOGA

The Path of Psychological Control

1

Perfection is within. The distortion of consciousness prevents its manifestation. Complete control over the mind-stuff is necessary in order for perfection to manifest itself.

THIS proposition is the primary concern of *raja yoga*. According to raja yoga, the obstructions to perfection are fundamentally the agitations within the mind-stuff. These are called *chittavrittis* (*chitta*, mind-stuff, and *vrittis*, ripples or waves upon it). By controlling the modifications of the mind, the yogi is able to control inner nature. Outer nature is then perceived to be only a manifestation of inner nature. Thus, perfection in raja yoga is the state of cessation of the agitations which obstruct the attainment of complete control over nature, inner and outer, individual and cosmic. Raja yoga teaches absolute control over the psychological and psychic forces within one. The main endeavour is to control the different modifications of consciousness. We must begin by controlling the grosser forms of mental agitation.

The system of raja yoga, the "kingly" or royal yoga, like all the yogas, has existed in India from ancient times. It may be called the "royal road" to perfection. A king controls his kingdom; we must control ours also. Our kingdom is our consciousness, controlling which we become masters of all nature. The highest authority on raja yoga is the ancient sage, Patanjali, who contributed the famous *Yoga Aphorisms*. This yoga is based on the Sankhya philosophy. God, as an all-powerful being to whom supplication may be made, is not recognized in this system. However, Patanjali says that God can be the subject of concentration and meditation. He prescribes meditation on God as *one* of the methods for the attainment of yoga, or highest union. I mention this to bring out the fact that in order to follow raja yoga one need not believe in or accept God.

A yogi was once asked what his profession was. Without hesitation he replied, "I am a farmer by birth and occupation."

"How much land have you?" he was asked.

He looked over his body with a glance and said, " About three and a half cubits." (A cubit is the measure of one arm, from the elbow to the tip of the middle finger, by which farmers in India measure land. Every person's height is about three and one-half cubits, measured by his own hand.)

Do you realize that the greatest property a man has is this "patch of land"—his mind and body? And that if he knows the art, he can raise a rich crop and gain the greatest assets one can attain in any field of endeavour? The yogi works his three and a half cubits and gains as his harvest the goal of life, which is perfection.

Yoga is that art of husbandry which teaches you how to cultivate this "land" and make the best use of it. It teaches you how to protect your property, clear the land, plough it, and prepare it for sowing so that you may reap the harvest.

To attain success in any endeavour a systematic method is essential. This is true in the case of raja yoga as well. Here there are certain practices and disciplines that help you attain the goal. When you acquire a patch of land, what is the first thing you do? You put a fence around it so that whatever crop you raise will not be damaged or destroyed by outside influences. You want to clear the title and keep out intruders. In the practice of raja yoga as well, the student has to adopt strong defensive measures.

I would like to especially draw your attention to one important point. It is for your own benefit and interest that you adopt these defensive measures. There is no external authority that compels you to do so. You, as a free being, of your own accord, choose to put a defensive wall around your "property." This is a very important point. When you yourself have chosen to put up a defensive wall around yourself, for the definite purpose of achieving success in yoga, you have gained one step towards the goal, for, to some extent, you have already asserted your spiritual strength. You have made a beginning, and to make a beginning is something.

In every religion there are certain commandments that are to be observed by its followers. But usually we do not find any psychological explanation for them. For that reason, people of this modern age rebel against the very word, "commandments." They might be convinced of the benefit and utility of some of them, but still they resent that some authority attempts to impose these commandments upon them. Therefore, the "thou-shalt-nots" in any religion are not very popular with many people today. Whenever we feel that something has been imposed upon us by an authority, and we have been denied free choice, we feel rebellious. I myself have a good deal of objection to this word "commandments." But, are they really commandments? They are principles, rules, regulations that have been handed down to us by experts, not by "authorities." With that evaluation, a rational, self-respecting "modern" should be able to accept them eagerly. In every religion these principles are nothing but the "defensive wall", that a novice puts around his field of life in order to raise the crop of spiritual perfection. In fact, if we do not build such a wall around us, we will be unable to succeed in any activity in any department of life.

Perfection in raja yoga means the attainment of that state of consciousness in which there is no bondage, no limitation, no imperfection of any kind. Consciousness in its pristine "form" or state is Brahman. As the yogi's aim is to transcend the bondage of limited consciousness, so his primary endeavour is to control his mind. The different obstructions to this goal must be analyzed and brought under control. To gain power over the lower self, one must start with some basic disciplines.

The entire system of raja yoga has been considered by Patanjali as composed of eight steps, so it is called *ashtanga yoga* or the "yoga of eight limbs." The eight steps are: *yama, niyama, asana, pranayama, pratyahara, dharana, dhyana,* and *samadhi.* We shall discuss all of these.

Patanjali discusses disturbances to the chitta under the first two categories, each of which comprises five disciplines. Under yama these are: the observance of non-injury, truth, non-stealing, continence, and the non-receiving of obligatory gifts. Under niyama the five are: cleanliness, contentment, self-discipline or austerity, regularity of study, and self-surrender to a higher power—God (if you believe in a God).

These ten preliminary disciplines are the "defensive measures."

We may call them the ten posts of a protective wall which the yogi builds around his field of action. I might mention here that these items form the very basis of ethics. For the first time in history, Patanjali established in the form of these disciplines a subjective standard of good and evil. Whatever actions and thoughts help to establish the calmness of the mind-stuff are to be considered good; those which distract from it are bad. That which takes us away from perfection is bad; that which brings us nearer is good. This is the yogi's standard of good and bad.

These practices must be understood, appreciated, and sincerely followed by every serious student of yoga. If he fails to practise these disciplines, his endeavour would amount to trying to fill a bathtub with water with the drain open. He may strive for perfection but if he is not particular about blocking the "drain," by means of these disciplines, he will eventually realize that it is all in vain, that nothing has been achieved. As a rational human being and sincere student, he must concentrate all his forces to check the wastes of energy; for these keep the mind in an agitated state. This must be done before he can proceed in his experiment with yoga.

The first discipline is non-injury, or *ahimsa*. You must discipline yourself so you will not injure any living being by thought, word, or deed. There are many aspects to this, both subjective and objective. The psychological aspect is that by doing injury to others, *your* mind is disturbed. The memory of having inflicted injury will arise in the mind like ripples on the surface of a lake, and frustrate all your efforts at meditation. If you hurt anyone, if you are jealous, or envious, rude or unjust to any being you can never enter the gate of yoga. A yogi must love and sympathize with his fellow beings. His life must be a life of service to all. Ahimsa has deep significance and a vast field of application.

Regarding the practice of non-injury in practical life, Sri Ramakrishna told a humorous story. There once lived a poisonous and vicious snake near a small village. He lived in a hole in a big tree and terrorized the villagers. One day a wandering holy man sat down under this tree and the deadly viper rushed out of his hole to attack him.

"Stop!" ordered the holy man calmly, "You have no power over me." Immediately, the snake lay still. "My son," the holy man continued, "why do you kill people for no good reason? I can understand a tiger or a lion killing for food, but with you killing is a pleasure more than a necessity. I'm going to cure you of this vice. I will give you a *mantram* which you are to repeat regularly. Promise me that you will not hurt anyone, for any reason whatsoever."

The snake promised and received the mantram from the guru, who then went on his way, saying that he would return later on to see the disciple. "Practise regularly," he told the snake, "and, remember, *don't bite!*"

Some months later the guru returned that way to see his new disciple. He went near the hole in the tree and called out the snake's name. But there was no answer. Again he called. Then the snake slowly crawled out of its hole. It was lean and emaciated. It hardly had the strength to move. The holy man was astonished to see this condition and asked the snake what had happened to him. In a faint voice the snake replied, "Revered guru, I repeated the mantram you gave me and meditated upon it regularly. I kept my promise to you about not biting anyone. But, the mischievous little boys of the village noticed the change in me. One day, one of the boys picked me up by the tail and whirled me round and round in the air, and then dashed me to the ground. Since then my body has been in this condition, for I have been too weak to go out for food. That is why, revered guru, you find me in this state."

"My son," said the guru, "it seems you did not fully understand me. I asked you not to bite anyone; I did not say not to *hiss!* In this way, you would have protected yourself."

So ahimsa has to be well-understood. It is not just a "namby pamby" relinquishment of all your rights. The practice of ahimsa is the first pole in the construction of your "defensive wall."

The second discipline is the observance of truth, or *satyam*. Truth should be followed with judgment and discrimination. Just making a statement of fact is not always truthful. The facts must be subjectively judged and understood in that light. Truth is often distorted through fear and selfishness. Overcome the tendency to distort truth; then the mind will not be disturbed by those waves of fear and selfishness, the subtle causes of the habit of lying. Observe truth, not only in speech but in act and thought as well. Truth is that which brings us nearer to perfection. Follow the truth in every gesture of your body. Saturate your whole being with truth so that your life becomes a living illustration of it. Then you will have taken one more step towards the realization of that perfection which is the goal of yoga.

Thirdly, the yogi must observe nonstealing, or *asteya*. Stealing means the misappropriation of someone else's property or right. This applies to both act and thought. It may be gross, emotional, intellectual, or spiritual. If you misappropriate the property of others, a wound will be inflicted on your consciousness. You cannot then expect to enjoy the depth of meditation. The non-recognition or non-acknowledgement of service done by others is also "stealing." Do not even appropriate the words of others without acknowledging the source. When Ramakrishna quoted anyone he would always mention, with reverence and humility, from whom he had heard the statement. In fact, Ramakrishna's life was the living example of all the disciplines of yoga.

The next discipline is *brahmacharya*, which means continence or the conservation of sex energy. The word can also mean "roaming in Brahman." For a person to exert his best in any line of endeavour, the conservation of energy is necessary. Brahmacharya is especially important for the student of yoga.

The benefits of continence are threefold: physical, mental, and spiritual. Behind the sex instinct is the instinct for immortality; if that energy can be understood and managed and converted into another channel, it will lead us towards the highest realization.

Human instincts and the dictates of a wayward mind are not always good. One shold be careful, however, not to be overly reactionary; this is almost as bad as indulging in excesses. Do not consider yourself "extra holy" merely because you avoid certain things. A student of yoga should learn to consider himself as neither a man nor a woman, but simply a human being. Sex consciousness is sure to bring a reaction from the opposite sex. Whatever may be the nature of the reaction, mental or physical, it creates disturbances of mind.

Medha, or brilliance of intellect, and a keen development of all the faculties are obtained by the conservation of sex energy. A strong body, a steady nervous system, and a brilliant mind, undisturbed by desires, are necessary requisites for the practice of yoga. Therefore, a student must rise above sex consciousness. This is what is meant by the practice of brahmacharya.

The fifth post in the defensive wall around the yogi's field of action is the non-acceptance of obligatory gifts, or *aparigraha*. This needs to be well understood. For one thing, if you accept gifts from people who expect something in return, do you think you will be able to maintain your independence? Will you be able to uphold fully the cause of justice where these people are concerned? The consciousness of obligation is always disturbing to the mind. Since gifts sometimes prove to be bribes, one has to be discriminating. Observe this principle: see that the giver has no motive except pure love. Secondly, see that the gift comes exclusively from the side of the giver, that it is given freely. The receiver should not expect anything. The acceptance of a gift greatly cherished in the form of a desire causes bondage. If there is no motive except pure love on the part of the giver and no expectancy on the part of the receiver, the gift will cause no bondage or difficulty.

Without mutual exchange this universe would be a desert. But guard your spiritual strength, your stamina. Cherish spirituality as a miser cherishes his gold, and let nothing diminish it. Spiritual stamina is affected by any gift or favour that tends to incur obligation. It is better to be prudent than to suffer. Gracefully avoid such situations. There is always a subtle exchange between the giver and the receiver, and vice versa, so beware of receiving gifts indiscriminately. In all contacts through gifts and favours always keep the eye of discrimination open. Do not be fussy or superstitious, but hold on to your discrimination.

There was once a yogi who had practised disciplines for many years. Once during his wanderings, he stopped at the house of a rich man and accepted his hospitality for the night. He saw a very costly article in the guest room. As he looked at it, a feeling of greed began to enter his mind. He could not control the thought. Suddenly he took the treasure and walked out of the house. Later, he thought: "What have I done! I have become *a thief*!" He immediately returned the costly article to the rich man and apologized, saying that he must have been in some kind of delirium. The wealthy man laughed at the incident and implored the yogi to continue as his guest. But he refused.

After some time, the yogi met another yogi who lived in that neighbourhood. He told him what had happened. The other yogi was not at all surprised. "Brother," he said, "I know the reason for it. Your system was contaminated by that man's hospitality. He has obtained his wealth by unfair means; every penny of his is dipped in the sweat and blood of innocent people. Through your acceptance of his hospitality, his dishonesty entered into your system. That compelled you to do this thing."

One should be very careful about the acceptance of gifts, favours, or hospitality from people. They have a very subtle effect on the mind.

The sixth discipline is the observance of cleanliness, or *soucha*. This means cleanliness, external and internal, physical and mental. As you know a great deal about physical cleanliness I will not speak of that. But here is an important point: cleanliness must be cultivated within, and expressed outwardly. Cleanliness is not something to bluff others with. No amount of external camouflage can disguise the inner untidiness. Do not try to practise that art of bluffing! A neat, pure mind is objectified in neatness and cleanliness of the body and clothes and in systematic and methodical work. Develop a neat mind and a neat habit of life.

In order to maintain mental cleanliness, allow the mind to register only the good things about people, not the scandalous. Remember that jealous, harmful, suspicious, and envious thoughts contaminate the mind. Gossip also makes the mind "dirty." We should train the mind to stay at home, and to ignore disturbing thoughts and influences. External cleanliness is the expression of that internal state of purity of thought and intention. They say, "cleanliness is next to godliness"—yes, mental cleanliness. Mental cleanliness means the practice of non-attachment. You cannot avoid becoming mentally unclean if you create attachments for things.

The seventh discipline is contentment or *santosha*. Show me a discontented and complaining person who has ever attained anything worthwhile. If one is always dissatisfied, one cannot make progress in any field. Some think that contentment hampers progress, but I have discovered that those who have achieved the most were anything but discontented. Those who are discontented are usually lazy and have no initiative. They do not achieve anything in any cause whatsoever. Do not think that contentment kills initiative. It does not. The tendency toward discontentment binds a person to his lower or material self. Contentment must be developed through discrimination. What is contentment? First of all, do not think that contentment depends upon the number of things you have at hand; it is a state of mind. Discontentment is a mental chaos that creates many ripples on the surface of the mind. Do not make a chaos of your life by generating discontentment inside yourself. Be cheerful and content with your present condition. Build on that. A dissatisfied mind finds no peace or poise. The perfection of yoga is impossible to attain for such a person.

The eighth item is austerity, or *tapah*. Many people shudder at the very mention of the word, "austerity." They think it means going without food or proper clothing or living in a dirty and shabby way. But were that the case, all the vagabonds of the world would be the best of yogis! The discipline of tapah may be defined as the practice of keeping evenness amid the dualities of life. Tapah is performed to gain the capacity to endure all dual conditions, such as prosperity-adversity, health-sickness, praise-condemnation, union-separation, and so on. You have to be able to accept "both sides of the coin" for peace and tranquillity in life. Mental poise is obstructed by our clinging to the pairs of opposites. By practising abstinence, evenmindedness is gained. Then it doesn't matter if someone throws a garland or an old pair of shoes at you!

A certain amount of abstinence has to be practised for any cause. Suppose you take up social service work and are called upon to render aid to people stricken by famine or flood or an epidemic. If you expect to have your meals and rest at regular intervals, do you think you can be a successful worker? In order to be a real worker you must discipline yourself to be able to go without physical comforts. That is what is meant by tapah. Discipline your body and mind so that, if need be, you can do without almost anything. That will bring you great strength. This body is a kind of machine that can be adjusted in any way you like. The ability to make such adjustments is absolutely necessary for one pursuing the path of yoga.

The yogi must cultivate a subjective mentality. We usually try to find the cause of disturbance in the external world, instead of controlling it from within, but the yogi is concerned with inner nature. Self-discipline should be observed in every function. Discipline the body, mind, and faculties so that the character may be strengthened. Purposely adopt a negligence in dress for some time and then, for the development of spiritual strength, endure the ridicule. Speech requires a good deal of discipline. "Let nothing be spoken by me that would hurt anyone." Practise this for six months. If you fail, punish yourself. Control of speech is essential for a student of yoga. Try to keep at least one day of silence each week. (However, let seven days be the maximum.) By taking constantly we close up many beautiful avenues of expression.

The control of speech is one of the most important disciplines of yoga. Try it. You will be able to detect many things that were not noticeable in that whirlpool of talking. Swami Premananda once told us: "You talkative fools! You talk nothing but nonsense! Let not your tongue talk; let your character speak." If you can quiet that tongue you will find that your character *will* speak. Talk just when necessary. Do not be a chatterbox. If we can control the tongue, the rest becomes easy.

At another time, Swami Premananda asked a group of young monks who were talking a lot: "Why do you buzz so much? You bees evidently haven't found the honey!" The bee buzzes loudly until it finds the honey in the flower. Then it concentrates on that and that alone, and is silent.

It is not as difficult to observe complete silence as it is to discipline the speech. The finer the mind the more susceptible it becomes to disturbing vibrations. For the yogi, austerity, or tapah, in all phases of his activities, is absolutely essential.

Regularity of study and steadiness in practice is the ninth discipline. This is called *swadhyaya*. Form a daily routine of practice and continue it regularly. Everything within is going on in rhythm. The force of rhythm consciously applied helps one to accomplish things without much effort. The rhythm itself will sweep you into the practice. This habit of regularity of study also brings a tremendous power of resistance. If you are not regular, tenacious, and steady in your pratices, if you are swayed and carried away by the slightest disadvantage, or if a little wind can blow you off your course, you will never achieve anything great. Don't be like a weathercock, changing with every breeze. Challenge all discomforts, obstacles, and difficulties. Tell them: "You may attack me on all sides, but you can never take me an inch from my footing. Even if all the world becomes antagonistic, nothing can stop my practice." You must have the determination of a hero. There are many people who do not get the desired results because they lack this virtue of tenacity and steadiness in practice. It is not so much the thing that is done as the regularity of doing it that establishes it as a part of your character.

One of the best examples of this steadiness in practice I have come across is that of a ninety-year-old lady in Benares. Every morning for over forty years she has sat and read aloud the whole of the Bhagavad-Gita. She has allowed nothing to interfere with her practice. She is not a scholar or a yogi; she calls herself an ordinary person of the world. But I have discovered qualities in her character that any yogi would be proud to possess. Recently I heard that one morning a monkey—monkeys are numerous and very mischievous in Benares—stole her spectacles. The old lady was quite perturbed because she thought that her long practice of the daily reading of the Bhagavad-Gita would be stopped for some time, until she could get another pair of glasses. But you will be amazed to know what happened. She found that by her daily practice for all those years she knew by heart its entire seven-hundred verses. Such is the power of steady practice!

If you can develop such steadiness for your practice, no matter what it is—whether it be reading from the Bible or from the Koran or other scriptures; prayer, repetition of a mantram; concentration or meditation or whatever—your success is assured. For twelve years, repeat the name of God five times every morning. If even that is done regularly, you will reap results.

The tenth and the last of these disciplines is the practice of surrendering oneself to a higher power. This is called *Iswara pranidhana*. Always maintain the attitude that you are being led by a higher power, call it God, the higher Self, or whatever appeals to you. Maintain the attitude that it is through the grace and kindness of that higher power that you are able to follow the prescribed practices and disciplines. Surrender your practice and the result of it to that power. If you retain the good results of your practices, they will bind you. Let all beings enjoy the results, if any; but do not look for personal gain.

Surrender the fruits of your practices to your highest Ideal. Take no credit for anything you achieve; and never try to measure your progress. Do not be like a person who is so anxious for the plant to mature that he digs it up each day to measure the roots! A Swami once met a childhood friend who asked him what he had gained by joining a holy Order. The Swami replied, "Brother, I have never totalled my account. I do not know how I stand."

As I mentioned, the ten perliminary disciplines of raja yoga which we discussed as the ten defensive measures that a "farmer" of yoga has to take for the protection of his three and a half cubits of "land," form the very basis of ethics; whether you are interested in practising yoga or not, the observance of these disciplines in your life will bring you success in any field of activity. It is needless to say that without observing these preliminary disciplines the student of yoga cannot proceed any further.

Next come the preparatory measures, which form the third and fourth limbs of raja yoga. These are the practices of posture or asana, and breathing, or pranayama.

2

AFTER building and carefully maintaining the ten supports of the defensive wall around his field of action, which we discussed in our last talk, the student then takes up the *preparatory measures*. Having decided of his own accord and for his own benefit to put a defensive wall around his "path of land," he now concentrates his attention on the "preparation of soil."

To continue our analogy of farming: the soil may not be in good condition; it may be rocky, stony, and covered with debris. It may not have the desired degree of fertility. What is done? The farmer removes the stones, deeply ploughs the soil, levels elevations and fills depressions. All this before he can think of sowing the seed. In yoga, this preparing for the sowing of the seed is done by the practices of asana and pranayama, posture and breathing.

In other words, the body must be made fit for the practice of yoga. A physically upset, disturbed, or weak person is unfit to practise yoga. Asana, the practice of correct posture, and pranayama, the regulation and control of breathing, are the preparatory measures which the student of yoga, at this stage of his progress, must begin.

Asana is the art of yogic posture. Through the practice of

correct posture, physiological, psychologial, and spiritual benefits are derived. By sitting in an upright position, we allow the organs to function best without obstruction. When we sit in a crooked position, there is a constant crowding, elbowing, and jostling going on within us. The internal organs are not comfortable; they are always quarrelling with one another. For that reason, they will not let us be comfortable. By observing good posture, circulation and digestion are also improved. So, even from the viewpoint of physical health alone, one should maintain good posture.

The man who stands or sits erect, chin up, looking the world squarely in the face, is psychologically more ready and able than others to meet emergencies. He has more confidence in himself, and is able to inspire confidence in others. Have you ever noticed that when you feel depressed or dejected you cannot sit erect? Your body naturally slumps into a crooked position. But if you receive some good news, you immediately straighten up. Do you know why? Uplifting news stirs a current within you which compels you to throw off the dejection. Thus, it follows that when you want to elevate your consciousness, you can do so by assuming a correct, upright posture.

The yogis say that there is a subtle energy, *kundalini sakti,* in a channel within the spinal column. By keeping the spinal column erect this energy is not obstructed. When one is spiritually uplifted, this energy rises like mercury in a thermometer. As this energy reaches certain levels, different states of consciousness are experienced. The practices which are intended to arouse that energy in the spinal column can only be undertaken when the yogi's asana or posture is perfected. Hence, for a student of yoga correct posture is absolutely essential. Even though the spine may be kept straight, lying flat or standing up creates certain distractions and disturbances, such as restlessness or sleepiness. Therefore, the sitting posture is prescribed for meditation.

The correct posture for yoga practice, therefore, is to sit in an upright position with the spine straight. In India, it is usual for people to sit cross-legged; they can do so for hours without discomfort. In the West, sitting on a chair with legs down will do.

Patanjali has defined posture as the capacity to hold the body still, in a composed and peaceful state, so that the maximum of success may be attained through a minimum expenditure of energy. One should sit in a posture which one can maintain for the longest period of time without feeling uncomfortable. Tense-ness defeats your purpose. For meditation, one should have a seat which is neither too hard nor too soft. The waist, chest, neck and head should be held in a straight line, the body being supported by the diaphragm. Place the right hand, upturned, upon the palm of the left hand which rests on your lap. The eyes should be looking straight out. There should be no feeling of strain, but one of ease and relaxation. Other eye positions are sometimes recom-mended, but for a beginner this relaxed position is the best.

If possible, sit facing the east. The reason for this is that the earth rotates in that direction and you gain a subtle benefit by facing that way. (In riding on a train, for instane, or on any moving body, it is *natural* to face the direction in which one is travelling.) If you cannot face east, then face north. There is a magnetic current always flowing towards the North Pole. In sleeping, follow the practice of the pullman porter, who always puts the pillow so you can sleep facing the direction in which the train is moving. All positive energy travels toward the North Pole. If we think of this energy as hundreds of balls being thrown south to north, over our heads, would it not be more comfortable to face north and let the balls be thrown over the back of our heads, than to face them? So, either for meditation or for sleep-ing, face east or north.*

There are many details in the practice of asana which have been developed by another branch of yoga, called *hatha yoga*. These practices are primarily intended for physical health and, for complete control over every muscle and nerve of the body. Many of the extraordinary feats we hear about are accomplished by adepts of hatha yoga. However, a student of raja yoga need not go into all of these, for hatha yoga tends to keep the attention more on the body than on the mind. The yogi's object is to eliminate body consciousness, for it interferes with concentration. If one is disturbed by body consciousness of any kind, one cannot concentrate the mind. When the physical shell is in an easy, comfortable posture we are least aware of it, and the mental

---

*Regarding asana, you might like to compare Patanjali's *Aphorisms,* II: 46-48, with the Bhagavad-Gita VII: 11-13. I should suggest that in your study of raja yoga you use as a text Swami Vivekananda's *Raja Yoga.* [*author*]

faculties are unhindered. Furthermore, the sincere student in spiritual life is not interested in extraordinary feats and exhibitions of power.

Pranayama has for its object the complete control of the vital energy in man. *Prana* means energy, *yama* means control. There are two aspects of pranayama: subjective and objective. Subjective pranayama means control of the vital and spiritual energy which is manifest in man. Objective pranayama means control of the inner prana in order to control outer nature. The laws of nature are outside our control until we can control them by subjective pranayama.

Prana is universal energy, cosmic power, "confined" within the microcosm. It is that force which is functioning behind every faculty, physical, intellectual, and spiritual. It is prana which is finding expression through all your thoughts and utterances. But do not think of it as being localized. Know it to be primordial, unmodulated, unmodified. There is but one cosmic energy and the human body is the greatest receptacle for it; the same energy manifests itself as gravity, electricity, and so on. In man, the mechanisms of the body are the conduits through which it flows. If that energy is controlled, anything can be accomplished. Remember that we do not use our own energy, but we "bottle" a little of the cosmic energy and use that. Life is the capacity of using prana; death, or inertia, is the inability of any conduit or mechanism to express prana. Prana seems to be modified according to its expression; but it is limitless and all-pervading.

The most tangible expression of prana is found in our breathing. While it is linked with this most vital function of the body, it is not the breath. Every expenditure of energy is registered in the respiratory system, so we may call breathing the "registration office" of prana. It is also the "controlling office." By regulating and controlling prana within himself, as expressed in his breathing, the yogi brings within his power the other phases of prana working in the microcosm. In that way he is gradually able to control his inner nature. Hence, a student of yoga practises to regulate and control the motion of his breathing. That, primarily, is what is known as pranayama.

In general, there are three important points to note about breathing: depth, rhythm, and the character of the breath itself. We all know that deep breathing is necessary for the health of the body. It exercises the lungs to their full capacity and vitalises the whole system. Correct breathing puts us, physically speaking, in such a favourable position that we are able to stay above many devitalizing influences of nature.

There are three benefits to be derived from deep breathing:

Physical: Besides exercising the lungs, deep breathing draws in more oxygen. Thus the body is strengthened. What does a man naturally do when he has to lift a heavy weight? He draws in a deep breath and holds, it, before he expends his energy. The deeper the breath, the more energy he draws upon. An energetic person is never a shallow breather.

Psychological: When one is mentally disturbed or depressed, breathing is shallow. Deep breathing calms the mind and keeps one above depression.

Spiritual: There is *something* which we draw in with our breath, for which we have no name. It is prana in its most subtle form, and we absorb this into every part of our body and mind. It may be called a divine force which sustains our body, mind, and soul. If one can practise deep breathing consciously for some time it will continue of its own accord and great benefits may be attained.

The second requisite for correct breathing is rhythm. Few of us realize what rhythm means in our lives. Rhythm is a fundamental principle that guides and regulates the universe. It also controls man. Anything done in rhythm creates a sort of harmony. Even rhythmic noise is not disturbing; but if the rhythm is broken, then comes chaos and confusion. If the noise of a moving train were not rhythmic, everyone hearing it could well be driven insane!

There is great psychological benefit to be had from the practice of rhythmic breathing. The first indication of anger in the body is the disturbance in the rhythm of our breathing. Have you not noticed that whenever you are upset your breathing not only becomes shallow but it loses its rhythm? On the other hand, when there is depth and rhythm in your breathing you *cannot* become upset. Try to become excited and angry, at the same time keeping your breathing quiet and rhythmical. You cannot do it. No burglar or enemy can ever enter the citadel of your body so long as the sentry of prana is guarding the gate, moving slowly and rhythmically. That is the key, the secret, of attaining peace and poise in life. Make rhythm the "home" of your breathing, just as the "home" of the needle of the compass is the North Pole. If a child plays with the needle of the compass, it may become unsteady; but as soon as it is released it will point towards home again.

The third quality of good breathing is its character. There are different types of breathing. The breath may flow like a silken thread or like a strong rope. Coarse breathing can be very disturbing, and is a sign of a crude mentality. In practising, to give depth to your breathing, be sure to retain the quality of fineness. Fineness in breathing is noiseless breathing. If your breathing is audible, analyze yourself and find out why it is so. Then rectify it. The character of your breathing may be changed by conscious effort. Correct faulty breathing. Try to make your breathing fine, deep, and rhythmical. That is absolutely necessary for the practice of raja yoga. Correct breathing is beneficial for everyone, whether or not he practises yoga. Whatever your object in life may be, whether you are interested in becoming a yogi or not, practise correct breathing for at least two years. You will reap a lifetime benefit. It is the finest of insurance policies. A generation of correct breathers could develop a new and greater civilization.

Before I give you a few of the breathing exercises of raja yoga, I should like to explain, briefly, the theory of the awakening of that potential perfection within, called the kundalini sakti. Kundalini means literally, "the coiled-up one." By the awakening of the kundalini is meant the manifestation of the potential power (sakti) which is in man.

The yogis believe that there are three channels in the spinal column for the passage of this energy. The one on the right is called *pingala* ; that on the left, *ida* ; and the middle one is the *sushumna*. Any agitation of the prana is registered in this spinal system. Ordinarily, the sushumna is closed, blocked as it were, at the bottom of the channel; as a result, the energy cannot enter it. This is what has been called the " sleeping " state of the kundalini, similar to the sleeping, coiled-up state of a serpent which, though dormant, has the potential of great strength. The objective of the yogis is to awaken this potential power, the kundalini sakti. When awakened, it travels up the sushumna, or the central channel of the spinal system, until it reaches the brain, at which place it unites with the Infinite. As it travels upwards it travels through six centres [*chakras*] which represent different stages of spiritual unfoldment. Symbolically, these centres are referred to as lotuses.

The full blooming of each lotus symbolizes the unfoldment of a certain spiritual state. The lotus is only a symbol ; you should not think that the yogis believe there are physical lotuses growing in the spinal column! The symbol of the lotus is beautifully representative of the unfoldment of spiritual understanding. The lotus bud slowly and gracefully opens its petals to the rising of the sun, symbolic of spiritual enlightenment in Hindu mysticism.

The first centre is the *muladhara*, located at a place corresponding to the base of the spine. The lotus of this centre is red and has four petals. With the opening of this centre, one gains the power of memory and control of the subconscious.

The lotus at the second centre is vermillion and has six petals. It is the abode of the animal self and is visualized as being located at the genital organs. It is called the *swadhisthana*. As this centre opens, we gain control over the animal forces which can be spiritualized and utilized for our spiritual progress.

At the navel is the third centre, the *manipura*, the " jewel city." The lotus is scarlet with ten petals. When this centre opens, we become convinced that worldly attainments will not bring us real satisfaction. At this stage we are able to examine their value and to throw them off, like clumps of earth.

These three centres are regulated, as it were, by a downward current, for there is always a pressure which threatens to throw us back into the " sleeping " state. Until the yogi is able to control these three centres he is not safe. He must struggle hard to reach the fourth centre. When he reaches that stage the spiritual current flows naturally upwards.

The fourth centre is at the place of the heart. The lotus is blue, with twelve petals. This is the *anahata*, meaning unagitated, uncaused. The opening of this centre brings one to the state of a causeless, universal love. One finds oneself present everywhere, manifesting universal love.

The fifth centre is at the neck; the lotus is smoke-grey, with sixteen petals. It is the state of complete purity. It is called *vishuddha*. It manifests in the personality of the yogi beauty, goodness, and truth. Everything he does reflects this.

At the place of the eyebrows is the sixth centre. The lotus is white with two petals. At this state the yogi unfolds absolute knowledge. He knows, though he *is* not yet *That*. This centres is called *ajna*, meaning "to know from near." Sri Ramakrishna described this state as one in which things are seen as though in a glass case. One knows what is inside of the case, but there is still a barrier.

The seventh state is above the six centres. The energy ot the kundalini, rising through the spinal column, at last reaches the *sahasrara*, the "thousand-petalled" lotus in the brain. This is described as a pure white lotus. There the kundalini "confined" within the system of man, merges with the Infinite in samadhi. That is the uniting of the self with the higher Self, the goal of the yogis. This cannot be described; it can only be *experienced*. The drop of water merges with the ocean. The potential perfection within you blossoms in the thousand-petalled lotus of infinite perfection and becomes one with it. This is an experience no one can tell you about. It can never be "secondhand." Each must experience it for himself.

Sri Ramakrishna used to try to tell his disciples about that state as he was entering it. He could talk for a certain time, but then the words were lost—in Infinity! When he *became* It, he could not *speak* of it. That is what is meant when philosophers say that Brahman cannot be known or objectified. It can only be *realized*. I might mention here that most of the yogis who reach that state are like the salt doll mentioned earlier, which touches the ocean and becomes one with it. They cannot return. Only the Avatars and the greatest spiritual giants can come back from that state.

In raja yoga, breathing exercises are intended to help awaken the potential perfection within, and to start it on its upward journey. There is nothing harmful or mysterious about the practices of pranayama, or control of breathing. They are proved, scientific processes. If properly followed by a qualified aspirant, they will bring the desired results. They should be done regularly, carefully, and *in moderation*.

First of all, do you know that we do not breathe clearly through both nostrils at the same time? At least, we rarely do. When the breath is flowing through the left nostril, in the case of a woman, and through the right nostril in the case of a man, breathing is considered to be most constructive for the exercise of positive energy. When the breath is flowing through both nostrils, the prana is said to be in a neutral state, which is good for meditation and rest. However, the breath usually flows through one nostril at a time. If you wish to alter this and shake off lethargy, and express constructive energy, do this exercise:

If you are a man, you will want to open your right nostril. Bend your left arm and press it against the left side of the ribs, inclining the body a little to the left. Close the left nostril with the thumb of the left hand and breathe deeply ten times, in and out. through the right nostril. You will find that it will open. The reverse is true for women.

Here are two exercises of practical   benefit to the physical system: (1) In a standing posture, turn the head to the left as far as possible. With the thumb of the right hand close the right nostril and breathe in through the left nostril, slowly and gently, to the fullest capacity of the lungs. Slowly turn the head to the right, hold the left nostril closed with the middle fingure and immediately open the right nostril and exhale through it slowly and gently. Then reverse the process.   This exercise will relax nervous tension. It is also very good to relieve a heavy, early-morning feeling. Do it five times before breakfast.

(2) Standing or sitting in any posture, purse the lips as though whistling. Without making any sound, draw the breath in thro ugh the mouth to the utmost capacity of the lungs. Then close the mouth, swallow, and exhale through both nostrils. Do this slowly and gently without any noise in your breathing. This exercise tends to improve the quality of the voice and relaxes the throat. It is good to do it in the open air.   Do this exercise five times every day, and in fifteen days there will be a noticeable improvement in you.

Now we come to other breathing exercises. In any position, sitting or standing, breathe in through both nostrils, irrespective of which nostril is most open. Breathe slowly and gently, exercising the entire capacity of the lungs, keeping the thought in your mind that you are drawing in with the breath the best of prana from the cosmic source. Without holding the breath, exhale slowly and gently with the thought that you are dispelling from your system all impure elements. As you breathe in mentally say the mantram, *Hum* which is a symbol of the thought that "I am drawing in and charging my whole system with the best of prana." As you exhale, mentally say the mantram, *Sah*, which is a symbol for the thought that "I am expelling from my system everything that is harmful or stale." Repeat this exercise in rhythm.

Before beginning meditation, sit in the correct posture and close the right nostril with the thumb of the right hand. Inhale slowly through the left nostril for four units (four seconds). Close the left nostril also, with the middle finger, and hold the breath for sixteen units, placing your consciousness at the base of the spine. Visualize the lotus of the muladhara centre and concentrate on the opening of the sushumna canal. Then open the right nostril and exhale through it for eight units. The rhythm is, therefore, 4-16-8. Reverse this process, each time concentrating on the opening of the sushumna canal as you hold the breath. For units, instead of counting, you may use the syllable *Om*.

In Sanskrit these three breathing processes are called *puraka,* inhalation; *kumbhaka,* retention; and *rechaka,* exhalation.

As the student progresses, the teacher may give him further exercises and guide him in their practice. However, without a qualified teacher one should not take up any further exercises or try to elaborate upon these given here. It might lead to disturbances of the physical or mental health of the student.

A word of caution. Do not think that because you practise a few breathing exercises you are superior to others. Beware of that attitude. Never let vanity take hold of you. The tail of the kite can become so long that the kite cannot rise. Do not carry along "tail" of vanity. It will hamper your progress. As you proceed in the practices of yoga, the ego should get smaller, not larger! Keep it under your control.

As regards the preparatory measures we have been discussing, there are two more important items: food and the occupation of time. These are referred to in the Bhagavad-Gita, Chapter VI, verse 17. In regard to your food, see that you do not eat to excess. Most people do. The average person also suffers from the wrong selection of food. Select food that is fresh and that has not lost its natural juices. Try to choose food that is not procured by causing injury to any living being. But do not bring up the question of carrots and potatoes! As long as we live we have to eat something. Life itself implies killing of some kind. But still I maintain that we should, if possible, live on food that is not obtained by causing injury to a living being. Conduct your own experiments. Break your habit once in a while. Do a little feasting and then a little fasting. Do not make a fetish of this discipline of food.

It is advisable to fast during certain days. According to the position of the moon there is an excess of fluid in the system on certain days; fasting on those days [ekadasi] will be good for you.

As regards occupation, in general, choose one that is in keeping with your ideas and ideals. That is, try to take up an occupation that does not clash with your desire to lead a spiritual life. You will have to use your own discrimination in this matter. The fact is, we should bring our occupation within the orbit of our spiritual practices. Know that by means of your job you are enabled to maintain yourself so that you may continue your practice of yoga, undisturbed by basic wants.

In your daily business contacts, you will find a wonderful opportunity for practising the disciplines of yoga. Apply the ten preliminary disciplines in your business life. Put them to the test, or rather put yourself to the test, and see how far you can carry them out. Even posture, to some extent, may be practised during your working hours. Also, the breathing exercises of a general nature may be practised. In that way, though you may be busy throughout the day, your job will not take you too far away from your spiritual life. This is true of your social life as well. And, I can assure you that your business and social contacts will be much more congenial, uplifting, and successful, even in a material sense. It is important, however, that you choose your occupation with discrimination.

As for leisure time, you can easily regulate your activities by making a routine for practice, study, and wholesome recreation. You can give your mind, and also your body, the discipline, food, recreation, and rest they require.

3

WE HAVE discussed the disciplines and practices that are necessary to place a student in a favourable position, or condition, for the attainment of success in yoga. To recapitulate: there are the ten preliminary disciplines that are basically essential for any success in spiritual life.* Then there are the practices of correct

---

* Noninjury, truthfulness, nonstealing, continence, non-receiving of gifts, cleanliness, contentment. austerity, study, and self surrender to God.

posture and breathing.

All these disciplines are intended to effect certain results in the character of the body and mind of the aspirant. But man does not stand alone; he is an integral part of nature and for that reason all his affairs, material and spiritual, are inseparably connected with natural phenomena. Consequently, yoga becomes easier of attainment for one whom nature has looked upon with favour, internally as well as externally.

In the consideration of this, there are three conditions necessary for a student of yoga to make any progress. First, there is that favourable disposition of his own nature, his body and mind; for that, definite practices and disciplines have been prescribed. These are the measures we have been discussing. Secondly, the student must have the favourable disposition of time. Thirdly, he must have the favourable mood of place or environment. I shall explain what I mean by these.

Subjectively speaking, there is no one moment in life ideally suited for spiritual exercises. You will find, of course, that there are certain periods of your life, even certain hours during the day, when your inner nature is favourably disposed to the practice of concentration and meditation. At other times, this is not so. If a student does not know the secret of availing himself of the favourable moments, he will have to do much hard, uphill work. Therefore, a student of yoga should analyze nature, both external and internal. He should find out the times when he feels the drawing in of his mental faculties and a natural and spontaneous hunger for spiritual exercises. When that "hunger" comes, he must do his best. As the saying goes, he must "make hay while the sun shines." It is something like the inflow of the tide into the rivers. When the tide comes, the rivers are full and there is a strong current. Know for certain that such a current will not last for long. When the ebb tide comes, it will be difficult for you to make much progress. There is a high tide in the flow of your life current. When that comes, practise and study diligently.

In the course of one's advancement, a time comes when one does not have to wait for any tide, when every moment of life becomes a favourable moment. Such a person does not have to depend upon time. His life is ever-flowing and ever-progressing. But before that stage has been reached, he has to take advantage of the favourable disposition of time.

There is another consideration of time, from the objective view-point. Irrespective of our personal tendencies, there are certain vibrations that control the whole of nature during certain periods of the day. Mother Nature is composed of three qualities [gunas]: sattva, peace, poise, equilibrium; rajas, activity the expression of energy in a dynamic way; and tamas, potential energy, or inertia. The external world is made up of these qualities. It is as if Mother Nature sprays her garden with various fluids to preserve its form and beauty. The influence of sattva, of peace, poise and equilibrium, is evident at certain periods of the day. Since meditation is a work requiring peace and poise, yogic practices can best be carried out during the calm periods of nature.

If you commune closely with nature you will find that there are these periods when nature enjoys tranquillity. These influence every one of its manifestations. Beasts, birds, trees, plants, flowers, rivers, even the very air—all seem, at those times, to enjoy tranquillity and calm. How can man, who has eyes to see and a heart to feel, help from throwing himself into that mighty current of inwardness?

Taking advantages of such a peaceful spirit in nature, such a quiet condition of your surroundings, you can achieve vastly better results than by practising at other times. For then, you have to work against the natural current. Suppose you are giving a musical performance. Will it be possible for you to achieve your best if the atmosphere around you is unfavourable? Suppose the audience is restless and unruly, noisy and inattentive? You would find it extremely difficult to express yourself well under such adverse circumstances. This is particularly true in regard to the practice of yoga.

There are four periods during the day that are considered the most favourable times for spiritual exercises. Technically they are called sandhyas, or junctures, when sattva, the force of tranquillity and peace, is more predominant. These periods are sunrise, midday, sunset, and midnight. The period of deepest tranquillity lasts for forty-five minutes during each period. That is, twenty-two and a half minutes before and twenty-two and a half minutes after the exact time of sunrise, etc. It is then that the whole of nature seems to be in a state of internal yoga. If you closely observe these times, you will find your inner nature urging you, as it were, to stop your mad thoughts for a while and enjoy the mood of contemplation. During these four periods, the student of yoga has the opportunity of availing himself of that favourable disposition of time when nature herself seems in a state of deep meditation. These periods also have power because of the collective thought-vibrations of advanced aspirants and yogis who are performing their exercises at those particular periods of time.

Many of you perhaps think it is impossible for you, for some reason or other, to practise at these times. It is unfortunate if you cannot avail yourself of these beneficial "currents." Try to take advantage of at least one of these periods. If it is impossible for you to obey this orthodox schedule, create by means of your own endeavour certain vibrations around you, so you can feel their effect at certain specified times. Choose your own time, but be punctual like a clock in keeping that time for your meditation every day. It is like having regular habits for eating and becoming hungry at those times. By the sheer force of association, create this favourable current around you, localized in time. Regularity is most important. If you practise at six o'clock today, seven tomorrow and ten the next, you will gain something; but you will be depriving yourself of greater benefits. Some days you may not feel like practising at all; you may experience a lack of enthusiasm. Your nature then needs coaxing and inducement. During those periods of dullness your acquired associations will help you, and external nature will also give you a "lift."

The third great factor regarding the favourable disposition of nature in yogic practices is "place." All places are not beneficial for a beginner. We have all been to beautiful places where our mind naturally withdrew from the world, where it felt inclined to soar high above the mundane. It wanted to go "home" to the Infinite. Sometimes, when you go to the beach (although we really shouldn't mention the beach as a place for contemplation!) try to find a secluded place near the lake or the ocean and look at that great expanse of water and sky. You will find your mind wanting to break all limitations. The inspiration one earns from such beautiful sights cannot be gotten by long practice in more ordinary places. Beautiful scenery exerts great influence on the mind. Such beauty spots are natural places for the practice and enjoyment of meditation.

A few years ago I was travelling through some of the national parks in the United States, among them the Grand Canyon. I left the crowd of tourists, found a secluded spot, and sat down to look out over the beautiful panorama, and enjoy the grandeur of the scenery. I forgot all about time; place-consciousness almost vanished. It seemed that I was alone, floating on the ocean of Infinity. How long I sat there I do not know. I received a rude shock when someone shouted, "Hey! You missed your bus! It left long ago. There won't be another one till tomorrow!"

My heart rebelled against all schedules and time-tables! Far better, I thought, was the free life of a monk wandering on foot, from place to place, alone and without ties, schedules, and appointments. I was reminded of a similar experience I had, but with a different ending. Some years ago I was at the Kamakhya Temple in the hills of Assam, in India, overlooking the beautiful Brahmaputra river. I will never forget that day of days in my life when I fed and feasted my inner being with something inexplicable. I think that was the best. meditation I ever experienced. There was no one on schedule to bind me to time or place!

When I see the beautiful places in this country, I am naturally reminded of similar beauty spots and places of pilgrimage in India. But I must tell you that the attitude of the people of the two countries towards these spots of magnificent scenery is quite different. Here, in America, there is much pleasure-seeking and merrymaking; there is a hubhub of excitement and noise. In India, an atmosphere of sanctity, reverence, and spirituality has been maintained for generations at these beautiful and holy places which are called *tirthas*. But I admit that we have pampered and extolled spiritual ideas and ideals at the cost of aesthetic and hygienic aspects. Nobody here is more conscious of that fact than I. I have often thought: why can we not have in India the same comfort, order, facilities, and cleanliness as we find in the national parks of America? But, if you come to those shabbily kept and unclean tirthas of India, and if you have the heart that feels, you will certainly experience a wonderful spiritual current around you. I might say that if there could be a harmony of the two—the wonderful spiritual attitude of India and the external orderliness of America—the results would be marvellous.

As things stand today, one cannot apply the same procedure here as one can in India in enjoying the beauties of nature in a meditative way. There is a story of an American boy who was studying yoga. He had read somewhere that it is good to sit for meditation on a rock surrounded by water. So he went down to the river, which flows through the city (he lived in Washington, D.C.) and found a big boulder with water surrounding it. With great joy he swam out to the rock and assumed the meditation pose. He was, however, not there very long when he was disturbed by loud voices. There, on the bank of the river, was a little crowd of anxious people with a policeman. The policeman called out to him in a loud voice, "Say! Don't you know you're breaking the law? What do you want to do, commit suicide? Come down from there, and get back here on the shore!"

So, in this western half of the globe, where people are always looking after someone else's business, one must take care. A corner of your little room may be safer than the "great outdoors"! Unless you can be sure of privacy it is better to meditate at home; though a place where you can gaze into the distance, where you can extend your vision into the infinite, is far better than being bound by four walls. However, if you cannot take advantage of a first-class opportunity with regard to the place for meditation, you will have to be satisfied with a second or third-class one. Create your own atmosphere in your own home. Set apart one room, if possible, to be used exclusively for your meditation. If that is not feasible, keep one corner of a room for that purpose only. Do not use that place for any other purpose. Keep it reserved for meditation alone. Keep a picture, if you so desire, of your highest Ideal in that place. That will induce your mind to withdraw from its usual orbit. Gradually, you will find that corner gathering a powerful vibration of spiritual forces which will help you a great deal. If you like incense, use it there. If you like flowers, put some there also. All these things form associations around your place of meditation.

In connection with the preparatory measures of yoga, which we have been discussing, there is another point to consider. In the analogy of agriculture and yoga, you will remember having to arrange for the irrigation of the land. In yoga this means the culture and development of genuine love and sincere devotion for your Ideal, as well as for all beings in the universe. If you are of a peevish temperament, if you create disturbances for others and others create disturbances for you—if such is your relationship with the world—you can never be a yogi. This is the test: do you feel a happy relationship between yourself and the rest of the world? If not, do not complain about the world. Do not say that you are surrounded by wicked and disturbing people, for that is not the reason. The reason is that you have not been able to develop yourself so as to be able to infect the atmosphere around you with love and friendship for all. You have to develop universal love, which will keep the "field" of your life in a condition ready to receive the seed. This is a virtue, a discipline, that should never be neglected. A peevish, complaining, and unsocial being can never be a yogi. You have to be all-loving. You have to be a living source, a channel, for carrying the message of love and friendship to all beings.

We hear much about the marvellous powers of yoga. These are called *vibhutis*. There are eight yoga powers which are known as *ashta-siddhi*. They comprise such powers as reduction into minute forms, power of expansion, levitation, the power to sway minds, and so on. But the most important "power" one can develop by yoga is that of ignoring them. There comes a time in the life of the yogi when the path forks. He must choose between the "Road of Cosmic Forces" and the "Road of Control of Consciousness." This is a very important stage of his life. When the fruit tree is fulfilling its destiny of bearing fruit it is bowed down humbly. Let the fruits of yoga appear on you, but follow the example of the fruit tree. Bow down! Do not crave yogic powers. The highest power is the power of peace, universal love, and divine knowledge. Other powers should be shunned. In the event of the appearance of unusual phenomena or powers, learn the greater power of ignoring them.

Real humility and sincerity of purpose, not the search for gain or powers, are necessary in any spiritual pursuit. Beware, also, of developing a fanatical attitude. There is a very apt poem written by Mira Bai, a saintly poetess of sixteenth century India. She was a queen who renounced her royal life to become a nun. I translate a few of the lines:

> If you think that you will become spiritual
> By washing and cleaning your body,
> Look at the fish.
> They ought to be your gods.

If you consider vegetarianism as the only way
To holiness.
You should become a follower of the donkey,
For he eats nothing but vegetables.
If you are partial towards fruit,
Make a monkey your god.
It is only by whole-hearted devotion and sincere love,
Says Mira Bai, that perfection is attained.

So do not be a fanatic. That only begets hatred for those who do not think as you do. And, remember, there is no short-cure to success in yoga. The ten preliminary disciplines, which are character-building, are at one end; samadhi is at the other. The order cannot be reversed. First things first!

I am reminded of a funny story. There was a young man who wanted to join a holy Order and practise yoga. He went to a monastery and asked to see the abbot. He told him that he wanted to be taken in as a disciple. The abbot asked one of the monks to show the young man around the monastery and explain to him what he would be expected to do if he joined the Order.

The boy was told of the various duties he would have to perform: rising early, meditating, drawing water, cleaning the rooms, working in the garden, and so on. He was shown the rooms of the initiates, with bare floors and walls, and hard beds. In passing, he saw nicer rooms, with softer-looking beds. He asked his guide, "Who lives in those rooms?"

"Oh, those rooms are occupied by the gurus," the monk replied.

As they passed the kitchen, the boy saw the plain food being prepared for the initiates and the young monks. Then he saw some trays of better food. "Who eats that good food?" he asked.

"That is for the gurus," was the reply.

"What do these gurus do?"

"They give instruction," was the brief reply.

The newcomer suddenly brightened and said, "Please take me back to the headman again."

When he came into the presence of the abbot, he said, "Sir, I have made a mistake. I don't want to be taken in as a disciple. I want to be a guru!"

But you cannot start at the top. You have to work your way there, slowly and patiently. How long it will take depends upon the effort you put into your practice.

After the preliminary disciplines and the preparatory measures have been established in your life, the seed of perfection will be sown. What is meant by sowing the seed? It means bringing out the potentiality which is already within you. After the majority of the preliminary disciplines of raja yoga have been attained, the aspirant draws a guru to himself. It is the powerful contact with the guru that brings out this potentiality within you.

Actually, it is not you who sow the seed. The seed was sown when the "land" was given to you. But it remained dormant because the necessary conditions for its growth were not there. When the required conditions are fulfilled, the seed will sprout of itself. But with practice we derive speedier results and, for that reason, mental practices or practices of concentration and meditation have been prescribed as *constructive measures.*

There are four steps to these measures. These one should practise sitting in the meditation posture, and after practising the breathing exercises which we discussed previously.

The capacity of human consciousness is infinite. In its pristine "form," consciousness is Brahman. Human or otherwise, consciousness is divine, is perfect. But there are limiting conditions that must be effaced before that perfection can be manifest. The mind, that part of consciousness which swings between the two poles of ascertainment and doubt, is always active. The mind is like a monkey drunk with the wine of pride, of ego consciousness. It is stung by six scorpions, our desires; it is haunted by five ghosts, the five senses. It is like a bag of mustard seeds scattered on a marble floor.

The aspirant in yoga must practise to concentrate his mind. Decide upon an idea, a form, or a concrete picture of your Chosen Ideal and try to fix your mind on That without thinking of anything else. You will find it very hard in the beginning to get the rays of your mind concentrated on one object. You will have to collect your wandering thoughts from all the different directions in which they are scatterd. Drive them from all sides, even as the shepherd gathers his wandering sheep. Centralization of thought is like the gathering of sheep by sending out dogs to herd them together.

The art of centralization, or pratyahara, means "to bring back to oneself." It requires regular and repeated practice to draw the mind together. One must practise regularly, every day. It is not to be attained easily; great effort is required. After practising pratyahara for some-time, you will be able to get a vivid picture of the object of your meditation. Your mind will become more steady; you will not have to work so hard to centralize it.

The second step is dharana, the retention or holding together of the collected consciousness for some-time. Having gone through pratyahara you have now gained some control over the mind and are able to focus your thoughts. However, it is difficult to hold it steady for any length of time. It moves to and fro. You have to hold the focussed mind on the object of your meditation. Do not let it get away. Refuse all other images. You may find that the object tends to become fogged. Keep the conception clear.

For example, assume you are concentrating on a lotus. First visualize the lotus in full bloom; then see it as being blue in colour. Then imagine that on the petals are letters of gold; expand your image, but do not let it become foggy; do not lose it. For this, you need practice and perseverance. When you have succeeded in holding the mind for some-time on the subject, without wavering, you will have reached the second stage, or dharana. The classic illustration of a steady mind is that of a flame of an oil lamp which does not flicker, but gives a steady light when it is in a place free from the wind.

Next is the practice of dhyana, or meditation. A continuous stream of "image-making" is called meditation. After fifteen minutes of such uninterrupted meditation the object drops from consciousness. Only super-consciousness remains. Or, you may say that meditation is like a continuous pouring of liquid from one jar into another. When you are in the stage of dhyana your mind will flow in a constant stream into the form of the *dhyeya*, the object of meditation.

Dhyana may be of two kinds, objective and subjective. When one meditates on an object, as we have just described, there is a subject-object relationship. This kind of meditation leads to a samadhi of a dual nature, called *savikalpa samadhi* ("with variation"). When no object is used for meditation, the Self, free from all modifications, reveals its own nature. This leads to *nirvikalpa samadhi* ("without variation," i.e., changeless). In subjective meditation, the endeavour is to remove from the mind all impressions and memories in order to prepare for the final revelation. (If the guest arrives and finds the room empty, he enters. Otherwise, he goes away.) We have to get rid of the upadhis, the vrittis that condition our consciousness in various ways.

When we meditate on the self within we draw the universe into ourselves. Or, we might say, in one type of meditation the self is expanded into the Infinite; in objective meditation the self is poured into the object, which becomes the All, becomes abstract Truth.

Samadhi, therefore, is the result of the preceding three practices of pratyahara, dharana, and dhyana. Samadhi means revelation. There are several different kinds of samadhi depending upon the type of meditation; I have mentioned only two.

When the mind casts its highest degree of concentration on an object, and holds it there for sometime, the reality of the object reveals itself. When the three factors of dharana, dhyana and samadhi function simultaneously in regard to any object, it is called a *samyama,* and the truth of that object is revealed.

Let me give you an illustration of these four steps of meditation. Suppose you want to create a powerful searchlight to illumine a particular spot. You must see that not a single ray of that light goes astray. It must be directed into one definite stream. That is what is meant by the first step of pratyahara. Then you have to put it on a base which can be so adjusted that the light can be fixed on any object. This process of fixing the light in a steady position is what is known as dharana. Dhyana is projecting the light for a certain length of time on the object, not allowing it to move a hair's breadth. Before such a powerful searchlight, things otherwise invisible are revealed. That is samadhi.

The "light" in the illustration is consciousness, or chitta. We began our practices of raja yoga with disciplines and exercises to remove the agitations, ripples and waves from the consciousness, from the mind. Having accomplished that we now have a powerful, steady searchlight, the *light of consciousness,* before which all is revealed. In the last analysis, there is only one chitta, one consciousness, but by the process of meditation the chitta which is "in the object," is revealed by the searchlight of "your" chitta. The subjective application of this is to turn the light on the"light" within yourself. The result is the highest illumination. This state of revelation of the subtle truth is the highest samadhi. Brahman, the inner reality of everything, subjective and objective, is realized. Consciousness vanishes and super-consciousness manifests. You realize that you are the One-without-a-second which is present everywhere, in every atom, from the highest to the lowest. You discover your own real Self, which is beyond death, beyond birth, and beyond joy and sorrow; which manifests itself in innumerable ways.

That is the stage of highest illumination. You know that you were always that divinity, that perfection, even when you were searching for it. You now know that you have always been carrying that perfection within you. You are the Self of all. The complete realization of that comes during the highest samadhi, which may be said to be the reaping of the harvest of raja yoga.

III

BHAKTI YOGA
The Path of Love

1

Man's emotion is the expression of a force within, which is perfection. Love is the positive expression of that force. By purifying the innate emotion of love within man, his inner perfection may be realized.

THAT is the proposition of bhakti yoga. The highest goal in bhakti yoga is infinite love, or God. Bhakti yoga regards man's natural power of love as a manifestation of the Divine within and teaches him to purify that love until it becomes omnipotent. By perfecting, magnifying, and extending the spark of love we have within us, we are enabled to realize God, who is infinite love. God is love; love is God. Manifestation appears out of love, is held in shape by love, and goes back to love again.

Devotion to God, to a higher, superhuman power, has always stirred the heart of man. The Vedas and other ancient scriptures of the world abound in beautiful sentiments, sometimes expressed in hymns which man poured out from the depths of his heart in adoration of, in awe of, and reverence for, a Being manifesting greater power than himself. In India, this primary urge to revere and to love a higher power was developed into a scientific procedure, a systematic method to gain realization, called bhakti yoga.

Therefore, bhakti yoga teaches the science and art of attaining perfection through the purification of man's innate love. It is science that teaches you to know; art that teaches you to do.

All emotion may be resolved into love. Love is the positive expression of that mighty force which is perfection. The negative reactions are anger, hatred, and so on. Instances of great heroes cherishing intense antipathy towards God, yet even then attaining Him, have been cited in bhakti literature. But, in all such cases, the ego-consciousness must be absorbed in the Ideal. In fact, it is the conclusion of bhakti yoga that any primary emotion, consistently cherished and intensified and carried to its logical conclusion, unfolds the inner, potential perfection in man.

The God of bhakti is identical with the Brahman of the Vedanta —one, universal, and infinite. But a *bhakta*, in order to cultivate his love, projects out of his consciousness a concrete, lovable God of his adoration, finite in nature, and calls it his *Ishtam*. Love is the recognition of one's highest Ideal, one's higher Self, in any object. When we recognize a certain ideal, we superimpose that on an object and love that object. When the highest Ideal, the higher Self, is projected and objectified in the form of a personal spiritual Ideal, it is called the Ishtam.

Supreme devotion to God, conceived as one's Ishtam, is what is meant by bhakti. Any object on which one exercises extreme love can be an instrument. But it is preferable to have a transcendental Being as the object of adoration.

A bhakta is taught to accept the personal Ideal, his Ishtam, and to love that Ideal until it absorbs his whole being. Hence, a bhakta's God, although a personal Deity or conception, is not an anthropomorphic conception of God. The theory of bhakti recognizes the psychological fact that in order to direct and cultivate his love, man needs an object in which to find manifest the highest ideal of his adoration. A bhakta makes God "in his own image," insofar as his Ishtam is a projection from within. It is his own private and relative interpretation of the universal Reality. Therefore, it is not to be discussed with or imposed upon others.

The Ishtam is "chiselled" out of the huge God of philosophy. The "stuff" is the same; you may make it any shape or size. There can be as many Ishtams as there are people. They are all personal readings of the Impersonal. No need to quarrel about the personal conception of God. I make my God and you make yours! I have not exhausted the "stuff" out of which gods are made. That is Infinite.

Let us take an example. A woman has four relatives: a father, a brother, a son, and a husband. Although she is one, she appears differently to each of these persons. She has a different relationship with each, since each regards her in a different way. And the woman? She is all those things for which she is loved.

Realizing that each man has the right to his own conviction, hold firmly to your own. Hold firmly to your own but be *ready* to say, "yes" to everyone. This tolerance of others displayed by the people of India is one reason why the Christian missionaries have not made more converts. The thirty-two million "gods and goddesses" of India are Ishtams, which the people have gradually come to accept, recognizing that each is a correct conception. The theory of Ishtam gives us latitude, gives us tolerance.

It is believed that the Ishtam is expressed through different incarnations. Hence, the need for a guru to determine the Ishtam of the devotee. The guru discovers the Ishtam for the disciple and gives him the mantram, or name, by which he is to address his Ishtam. With love and faith the disciple repeats the name of his Ishtam, the name of God. Gradually, by the repetition of the mantram, many things are revealed to the disciple. The highest realization is brought nearer and nearer to him. Suppose that a casket of jewels has been sunk in the ocean and you want it. Suppose we say that it has been sunk in the Atlantic Ocean. And that is not a bathtub! You want it, but you do not know just where it is. When your yearning for it reaches a certain state, the guru comes. He is an expert. You are standing on the shore of the ocean and he dives in, finds the casket, and attaches a chain to it. When he comes up out of the ocean he gives you the end of the chain and says, "Pull! Then you will get hold of the casket of jewels."

The mantram is a link in that golden chain that is tied to the precious casket of "jewels" sunk in the ocean of Infinity. By repeating the mantram, that is by pulling, link by link, the casket of realization comes nearer and nearer to you. You go on pulling, not knowing how long the chain may be. It may be short or it may be very long. But with faith and the intensity of love, you go on pulling, link by link, with the hope that the next pull may be the last!

In considering the Ishtam of the disciple, the guru takes into account the disciple's past. He analyzes the tendencies in the disciple. He may have talks with him, may make a few "experiments," and may also meditate in order to discover the correct Ishtam for the individual.

One-pointed devotion to the Ishtam is absolutely necessary for a bhakta. This is called *Ishta-Nishtha*. We shall discuss this a little later. Philosophy, learning, the power of reasoning, logic, and so on, are like the tusks of an elephant—both for show and for protection. But Ishta-Nishtha is like the elephant's set of teeth which he uses to eat his food to sustain and nourish himself. Polish your "tusks" of philosophy and learning and be proud of them, but realize that the aim of life is to nourish and sustain your true Self.

In yoga the aspirant is called an adhikari, a fit recipient, a container. The adhikari of bhakti yoga has been described in the Bhagavad-Gita in Chapter 12, verses 13-20. The main characteristics of a bhakta are purity, loyalty, trust, and spontaneous devotion. There should be no "ifs" about his devotion; it must be whole-hearted. There are three types of adhikari: fast, medium, and slow. The "fast type" can understand the intentions of the scriptural injunctions, as well as the teachings of the guru, even without being told. He can grasp instructions as soon as they are presented to him. The "medium type" is one who understands and assimilates the instructions when they have been repeatedly explained to him. The third, or "slow type" is one who does not understand, though he is told over and over again. He fails to assimilate the teachings for a long time. All three of these types are sincere. They are all struggling to advance, but some have to struggle more than others.

Men are not born of equal calibre. They should, of course, have equal opportunity; but they are not "born equal." Each has behind him a storehouse of karma that directs his present life. It shows up as tendencies, talent or lack of talent, capacity for understanding, and so forth. Dry firewood catches fire quickly. Likewise, some adhikaris can easily understand the teachings and incorporate the disciplines into their lives more readily than others. But you cannot set fire to a banana plant. It only smoulders and raises a screen of smoke. Sri Ramakrishna once said of someone: "What can I do with him? He is like the trunk of a banana plant. I cannot set it on fire even if I try; it will only smoke and smoulder. His eyes will be sore and so will be mine!"

Human beings are characterized by tamas, rajas, and sattva, one or more being prominent in the character. Each must follow the path according to his own nature. In spiritual life it is not necessary or advisable to try to keep up with someone else. Don't waste your time trying to figure out what someone else is doing. It is not necessary to keep pace with anyone else.

In dealing with the emotions, as we are doing in bhakti yoga, we find that some people are overwhelmed by a sudden and strong devotional feeling, but then are quick to lose it. They are like flowers that bloom only for a day, and then fade. Others are like the giant redwood which grows slowly and steadily, but never stops. There is really no way to expedite bhakti except to let it grow, to allow it to grow by removing the obstacles to its expanding nature.

After an adhikari has formed an unshakable comprehension of his Ishtam, he sinks, like an oyster, into the ocean of *sadhana*, or spiritual practices, and slowly and patiently develops the pearl of his *bhava*. Sadhana means "practices or disciplines"; bhava literally means, "state of being." In the literature of bhakti it means the attitude of an aspirant towards his Ishtam, in the form of a consistent relationship.

If you were given the power to make a form which was absolutely perfect, expressing your highest Ideal in that shape (as you would mould a figure in wax) the emotion with which you would adore it would be bhava.

Bhava should be strictly personal and confidential. Do not interfere with others by trying to impose your ideas and ideals upon them. In some instances, bhava develops from one stage into another, like a bud blossoming into a beautiful flower. However, a good deal of practice and much discipline are necessary. Don't simply be a "time-server."

Bhavas are innumerable, but they have been classified under the following categories:

Santa bhava—The relationship of transcendent awe and admiration towards an all-powerful Being.

Dasya bhava—The attitude of a servant towards his master. The spirit of humble service from a distance.

Tata bhava—The attitude of a child towards its parents. (In bhakti yoga God and may be looked upon either as a masculine or a feminine Entity.)

Sakhya bhava—The attitude of a friend towards a friend.

Vatsalya bhava—The attitude of a parent towards a child.

Madhura bhava—The attitude of a lover towards his or her beloved.

Any other strong, consistent emotion will lead one to the goal. *Darsana*, a clear perception of the Ideal, follows the establishment of one of the bhavas. A bhava controls one's life-current.

Sadhana is the systematic practice one follows in order to develop a bhava. It presupposes a constant fighting for some time with obstructing agencies. What are these obstructing agencies? For the most part they are all due to the ego, to a wrong conception of the ego. Bhakti yoga teaches absolute self-abnegation. It leads man's natural love through steps and stages of self-purification. It is dualistic to start with, but in the end brings the realization of Oneness, by merging the I into the Thou. When love is purified and well-regulated, the God of Love is revealed as the Ishtam. Love is a psychological phenomenon and by the cultivation of it into its highest form, the Divinity is revealed. Love is the bridge which connects you to your higher Self, with the conception of your highest ideal of beauty, power, and perfection. Love is nothing but the recognition of your highest ideal in the object of your affection, thereby establishing a bridge of communication to your higher Self.

Purification of love is necessary, for love in the ordinary sense of the word is self-seeking.

What are the steps one has to follow in order to reach divine Love? Let us spell it. L-O-V-E. *L* stands for *longing,* the longing for the Divine. Without this longing, no progress can ever be made. The letter *O* means *Oneness.* What is it the bhakta longs for? Oneness with the divine Ideal. *V* stands for *vanity,* for selfishness, the wrong ego-consciousness. What thwarts us in realizing this Oneness? Nothing but this. All the rituals, disciplines, and other stages through which a bhakta must go are intended for one purpose only, to eradicate wrong ego-consciousness in the bhakta. *E* is for *ecstasy,* which is the culmination of the practices of bhakti yoga. When you use the word "love," remember what it really means.

Technically, there are three stages through which a bhakta must pass before he attains the realization of his bhava, before the bhava is established and darsana (seeing the Ishtam) is reached. These are:

Vaidhi bhakti—The word vaidhi is derived from the Sanskrit root *vidhi,* which means law, injunction, formality. This stage is regulated by many do's and don'ts—rituals, disciplines, and so on. It is the stage of obedience to regulations.

Raganuga bhakti:—This means love following attachment. At

this stage love is expressed in the form of demands.

Prema bhakti—This is the state of "not I, but Thou," when there is absolute negation of self, and love alone exists. Prema leads to the consummation of bhakti, or *bhava samadhi*, the goal of bhakti yoga.

The rules and regulations of vaidhi bhakti are compared to a fence around a wayside tree. The fence does not contribute to its growth, except in a protective sense. The tree may even feel that it is being hindered. If it could talk the little tree might protest against it. But we must have the fence of disciplines until we are sure we do not need it.

The flower first appears on the gourd plant; then it dies, and the fruit develops. The decay of the flower indicates the development of the fruit. The flower must not be injured because of the fruit. Forms and rituals are the flower; love is the fruit. Rituals in bhakti yoga must be followed patiently in order to "fall in love" with God. (But, then, why should we say "fall in love"? We *rise* in love!)

Behind the formalities of our worship, attachment develops. Then the attachment becomes the motive-force. Vaidhi matures into love-following-attachment, or raganuga bhakti. So forms and formalities become secondary. It is one's own sense of adoration that prompts formalities at this time. Before, it was forms that guided the activity.

In ordinary affections the two stages of vaidhi and raganuga are followed, but we do not reach prema. We are not constant enough in our love. Our love always has too much self in it. A mother's love is the greatest manifestation of ordinary, human love.

Bhakti is an organic, psychological system of growth and it must follow its own course. You cannot really expedite it. Let the growth be normal and the fruits will appear of themselves. We must wait, with *willingness,* for the fruits of bhakti to appear. Sri Ramakrishna told this story:

Narada, one of the immortals, was, in his freedom, wandering about before returning to heaven. Passing an ascetic who was seated by the roadside, Narada spoke to him. When the ascetic learned that Narada was on his way to heaven, he requested him to ask the Lord how much longer he must wait for illumination. This Narada promised to do and proceeded on his way. Soon he came to the house of a devotee named Shanta Ram. Shanta Ram was singing and dancing in joy, full of selfless love for the Lord. He also requested Narada to ask the Lord how much longer he must wait.

Time passed and again Narada, on his travels, came that way. By this time, the ascetic was nearly covered by an ant hill. He anxiously asked Narada what the Lord had said. Narada told him: "You must wait just three more incarnations."

"Three more incarnations!" cried the ascetic. "That is too long! After all this renunciation, meditation, and these austerities, and *still* I must wait for three more incarnations! I give up!"

Narada then went to the house of Shanta Ram and delivered the Lord's message to him. "Shanta Ram," he said, "the Lord has said that you must wait for as many incarnations as that huge tree has leaves." And there were many leaves on that tree!

"So soon!" exclaimed Shanta Ram, and leapt with joy. "Oh, the Lord is so gracious to me!" The Lord heard him, and seeing his devotion and patience granted him immediate illumination. It was his willingness to wait for the fruits of his devotional practices that won him the prize of freedom.

In the curriculum of bhakti yoga you must first graduate in these subjects:

1. *Niyama:* The niyama disciplines are the same as prescribed in raja yoga. They are part of the fence you put around your little, tender plant of love for God.

2. *Nishtha:* Nishtha is that condition which makes you adhere to certain forms and rituals, not allowing any circumstance or human influence to stand in the way of your following them. When niyama becomes steady it is nishtha. Nishtha is a kind of dogged persistence, a "bulldog tenacity." Fanatics have it. Nishtha makes it possible for you to "hang on" to your practices with tenacity. This force, alone, can lead you to the goal.

3. *Upasana:* This means to stay near the object of your worship. This may be accomplished through all your activities. In the stage of vaidhi bhakti it is done by following four practices in particular: *puja, japam, smaranam,* and *dhyanam.*

Puja is the ritualistic worship of your Ishtam. Do all the rituals as if he were present before you. Consider the Deity as a member of your intimate family and worship and serve him. Consider him as your master and always work for him.

Japam is the repetition of a mantram, or, the name of the Ishtam. Repetition of the Name is a great purifier. Repeat it as often as you can. Traditionally, some word symbols have been associated with certain ideas, and by constant use these have gained power. As you repeat the mantram, which is your own, you create a vibration of spirituality around yourself. Repeating the beloved's Name is necessary for success in bhakti.

Smaranam means constant remembrance. Stop occasionally in what you are doing and punctuate your life with a little remembrance. Remembrance, harmonizing all the forces of your being, becomes the undertone of your life, and life becomes a symphony.

The hand of the compass always points north. Let the Name be the North Pole of your life and your mind like the needle of the compass. That is remembrance.

At wedding feasts there was always a man whose duty it was to see that all the lights were kept lit. He would move from one light to another, pouring more oil wherever necessary. He also would sit and talk with the wedding guests. But his mind was always on the lights. That is remembrance.

The maidservant tends to the children of her master, calling them affectionately, "My Hari, my jewel," and so on. But all the time her mind is on her own dear children in her far-away village. That is remembrance.

A man has a toothache. He may go about his business attending to urgent matters, but his mind is on his toothache! That is remembrance.

Cultivate remembrance of your Ishtam.

Dhyanam means meditation. By developing smaranam, one is able to meditate successfully on the Ishtam. Meditate upon your Ishtam on the lotus of your heart, or as instructed by your guru. The Ishtam is the master of the body, mind, and spirit. Concentrate all your faculties on him. Let your inner eye feast upon the beauty of the Ishtam within. Make your body the actual temple of God. Meditation on the object of adoration purifies love. One gradually takes on the qualities of the object of meditation.

4. *Dinata:* Dinata means modesty, humility; but not the humility that comes from thinking: "I am a good-for-nothing." When you are conscious of a great power within you, you become

really humble. Dinata is based on the realization of something very great. It is a great purifier of love. Be ready to give honour and respect to all. Attain this virtue of dinata. Strength, not weakness, comes from dinata. Be ready to be trampled on like a little blade of grass. Be like a fruit tree that gives fruit in return for a stone. Be like the tree that gives shade to the woodcutter even while he is chopping it down.

As soon as the name of Nag Mahashaya (a householder disciple of Sri Ramakrishna) is mentioned to someone who knows his life, the most exquisite picture of dinata comes before the mind. It was said that the Divine Mother tried to bind Nag Mahashaya with her rope of maya. But he became smaller and smaller, more and more humble, and she could not find anything to tie the rope around. She tried to bind Naren (Swami Vivekananda) in the same way. But he grew bigger and bigger, his self expanding into the infinite. Her rope was never long enough to tie around him!

Once Swami Shuddhananda was visiting the Patna Ashrama when I was there. When it was time for the scripture class, I requested him to take the class. I felt reluctant to do so with a senior Swami present. But he would not do so. Instead, he sat very modestly among the students while I conducted the class. That is an example of dinata, the humility practised by great souls.

Sri Chaitanya emphasized dinata and japam. "Be humbler than a blade of grass; more patient than a tree. Always give honour to all; want nothing for yourself."

5. *Seva*: Seva means service; rendering service to your God as a form of worship. Your God is the recipient of your devoted service. Doing social service work in hospitals, and so forth, often begets an attitude of pity. Do not, even subconsciously, think that you are doing anyone a favour. When some of these club women talk about their "charities," I feel like saying, "Mother Earth, crack, and I will enter!"

Consider yourself fortunate to have an opportunity to serve your beloved God personally. The sales clerk's "What can I do for you?" is the wrong spirit. Do not think like that. Even if you do not see your God, you see His children. Serve them. If you are a teacher, think that the students are God manifesting Himself before you.

6. *Atmasamarpanam* means self-surrender to God. Rely on the Deity. Hold on to the hand of the Deity and let the Deity hold on to your hand. Then you will not slip and fall; your path will be much easier than otherwise.

Vaidhi bhakti, as you see, is ritualistic. These rituals must be followed by a bhakta in order to strengthen himself and to cultivate his love for his Ishtam. Rituals are the mode which you follow in order to enjoy the object of your devotion.

2

IN THE first talk I mentioned the bhavas or different attitudes a lover of God may have for his Ishtam. I should like to contribute a little background to this, as it my sound new and strange to you in the West that God can be adored through different relationships.

Of all the peoples in the world, the Hindus alone have discovered the secret of loving God as a mother or child, friend or sweetheart. To them God is not a person, but a Principle which may be viewed from many angles. The Hindu is an abstract thinker. He puts the ideal first and then the person; the thought and abstract principle first, and then the creation of gross matter. To him the body does not *possess* a mind and a soul; rather, the soul gives birth to the mind and body. Persons have value so long as they typify a principle.

Throughout the length and breadth of India, the "Krishna Ideal," in its many aspects, is worshipped and idealized even today. The Hindus can reject the person of Krishna any moment, but the Krishna Ideal is the very life of their lives. It forms the very foundation of their being, and it embodies a great deal of the history of their civilization. In order to understand the Krishna Ideal we must proceed gradually from the concrete to the abstract; the personality will be eclipsed by the radiance of the magnificent Ideal. In Sanskrit this process is called "arundhati darsana nyaya" or the showing of the arundhati, a small, nearly invisible star. We have mentioned this process earlier. As you might recall, the teacher first points out to the student gross objects, then the bright stars, then the others less distinct, until at last he succeeds in pointing out this almost invisible star. Similarly, the mind of the spiritual student must first be drawn to some person in whose character the Ideal is typified. Gradually, as the mind develops the power of grasping the abstract truth, it can do away with the person and cling to the Ideal.

An eminent writer once wrote, in appreciation of the Hindu psychology of bhakti, that the Hindus have taken down the stern God of justice of Christian theology from his throne in Heaven and given him a place in their homes as Mother Friend, Child, or even as Husband or Sweetheart. God, in order to be a beloved God, must come down from his exalted position as a punisher of sins. He must be near and dear to us. This ideal of a sweet God, a lovable god, a playmate God, has been typified in the Hindu religion in the personality of Sri Krishna, whom we find tending his flocks on the banks of the Jamuna, playing with the cowherd boys and charming everyone with the sweet music of his flute, which symbolizes the attraction of divine love.

The poet of the *Bhagavata* depicts the child Krishna as the personification of the love aspect of Brahman. The principle underlying the phrase, "God is Love and Love is God," is found admirably illustrated in the personality of Sri Krishna. The poet is ecstatic in describing in fullest detail the wonders and miracles wrought by the universal principle of love.

In the person of Sri Krishna are embodied three special aspects of love, sakhya, vatsalya, and madhura, or the love of friend for friend, mother for child, and that of a maiden for her beloved. What a charming picture of ecstatic love has been depicted by the poet in describing the various phases of love represented in the character of Krishna! There are many scenes of sakhya bhava, the love of friend for friend, which the cowherd boys enjoyed with Krishna in Brindavan. Even the cows and calves were fascinated by him and would not go to graze until they heard the maddening sound of Krishna's flute. His smile, his touch, his mirth, his songs, the divine melody of his flute—all added sweetness to everything concerning the lives of his friends and companions and even of the birds and beasts of the forest of Brindavan.

How tender and natural is the picture of the love of Yasoda, the adopting mother, towards her Gopala. That was the endearing name she called Krishna. He is depicted as a charming child with exquisite personal beauty, full of mirth and sweet mischief-making. In one scene the young imp is seen stealing butter and cream from his mother's kitchen. I once heard a missionary say, "Your Krishna was a thief, yet you still worship him as God!" I cannot but pity a religious teacher unable to conceive of the lofty, noble, and sweet beauty of the Krishna Ideal. But how can he do so when, most likely, he views God as a frowning, wrinkled old man (perhaps like the magistrates of our criminal courts) sitting with heaps of paper beside him that record the sins of men and for which he metes out various punishments; how can such men understand the lovely and charming Krishna Ideal? Krishna is a fascinating, lovely child who attracts your love more than your reverence.

Crowning all are the love scenes of Radha and Krishna. The subtlest of feelings, the tenderest, finest, and sweetest of love that transcends body-consciousness, that love in which every consideration of earthly existence wanes into nothingness—that love has been depicted in the mystic and psychologically subtle relationship of Krishna with the charming girl, Radha. If love at its highest culmination, in its extreme form of selflessness, in its yearning to the utmost degree for the ultimate reality—if these could be given form and depicted as a person, such love would surely be embodied as Sri Radha of Brindavan. Radha is divine. She is beyond the comprehension of gross minds and intellects, which know nothing but enjoyment of the senses. The most exquisite gem of purest lustre, in the story of Krishna, is Sri Radha. She is so fine and so delicate that she cannot bear the lecherous breath of the worldly-minded. Madhura bhava, or the love for God as the Divine Lover, is too delicate to be handled by those who live in their senses. It begins where the senses with their sense-objects are not.

Sri Krishna of Brindavan, the embodiment of love, is the personification of the whole history and psychology of love. Who cares for the person, Sri Krishna, if the divine principle can be realized in our thoughts and actions? Even today, if one ideal could be named which receives the highest worship in the hearts of Hindu men, women, and children, it is the Krishna Ideal.

Krishna is still playing on his divine flute. Shut your outward senses, look within, go deeper into the innermost recess of your heart and float on the bottomless waters of unselfish love, and you will surely hear it and become immortal!

Love in any form when exercised for sense pleasure is lust, which degrades the soul and leads it to bondage. When that very same love is not conscious of the self and wants nothing in return, it merges the subject into the being of the object loved. That is prema, or divine love, which liberates the soul from all bondage of the flesh and makes the lover one with the principle of love—Brahman.

Sometimes people ask, "Did Krishna really live, or is he just a mythological character?"

My answer is this: Although there is no historical evidence regarding the advent, life, and teachings of Sri Krishna, we receive a thorough knowledge of the *ideal* for which this great man lived from the Sanskrit epic, the *Mahabharata*, the *Srimad Bhagavata*, the *Harivamsa*, and other *Puranas*. In fact, Krishna is the hero of all these; the teachings contained in them centre on the ideas and ideals exemplified in his character.

Today, in our research of history, we give too much importance to personalities and not enough to the ideals personified in their characters. We are satisfied when we can find evidence of the dates and places of birth of such heroes. But with the ancient Hindu historians, if I am allowed to call the compilers of the Sanskrit epics by that name, the ideals came first; the personalities were considered as illustrations of those abstract principles for which they stood. It is for this reason that the personalities of the Hindu epics seem to the modern mind to be wholly mythical, without historical basis. But it seems to me that if those "mythical personalities," as we may call them, can exercise such great influence in moulding the destiny of a race, if the ideas and ideals underlying those great characters can inspire and guide the lives of millions of people for thousands of years, then they are more real and worthy of respect than so-called historical personalities.

Now let us return to our discussion of the practices in bhakti yoga.

The state of raganuga bhakti, as I mentioned before, is the state of love that follows attachment. This is a turbulent state, filled with intolerance, jealousy, anger, and impetuosity. It is self-imposing, domineering and characterized by wilfulness. (The baby wants to pet the cat, whether the cat is willing or not!) At this stage, love is disturbing, desiring its own satisfaction, and jealous of others. The attitude towards others is often: "The king smiles on *me!* Who are *you*?" It is the period of *I* and *mine,* and suffering is caused when that consciousness of *I* and *mine* is being knocked out of you! It is the real fire test. When you have a piece of gold mixed with some extraneous matter you first hammer it to eliminate the dross, to get the pure gold. Through this hammering, some of the dross is disposed of. (If after a few blows nothing is left, it was not gold, *not love*. It was just "bargaining.") Then you scrub the gold. The constant friction cleans it some more. Then you put it into the fire. If, after that something comes out, that is pure gold pure love. Nothing will tarnish it. There is no more dross to be taken out of it. Do not speak of your "love" until these processes have been gone through.

In this state of raganuga, the attachment is more to the ego than to the Ishtam. The quality and the quantity of your love require to be changed. The fire of selfishness must be 'rowned by gallons of tears! Sacrifice the beast of selfishness before the altar of your love.

Raganuga is more natural and spontaneous than vaidhibhakti. It has a great deal of the mind's action and reaction in it. You are entering into a mental region of the discipline of the ego, more than the region of disciplinary action. For that reason, this stage is a little more troublesome. There is more disturbance. In fact, the state of raganuga is a very, very difficult one. It is a process of growth of the I, and then the merging of the I into the *Thou*. And in this process the *I* has to undergo a lot of cleansing.

When a bhakta becomes really attached to God, God becomes "smaller" than he used to be. The huge transcendental personality which you previously stood in awe of, which you gaped at in wonder as a worshipper from a distance—that God becomes nearer to you. The attitude of "ownership" towards Him becomes dominant during this period. The attitude becomes: "God is *mine*. I am the caretaker of God. He must do what I want him to do!" and so on. You want to own that God, as you might own anything material. And the subtle characteristic feature is that in this stage you seek mostly your own pleasure and happiness. You forget that the distinguishing feature of true love is that you wish to give and not to accept. During the stage of raganuga one loves in a selfish, demanding, possessive way. The self, the *I am*, becomes a little pampered, at this stage. The devotee wants everything for his own benefit. Avidya, ignorance, has so many offsprings. The

I am, in a limited sense, begets attachment, which leads to pride, anger, jealousy, and so forth. This results in sorrow and suffering. If you persist through that flood of sorrow and suffering, the *I am* consciousness will be cleansed and love will flow in a different way.

Bhakti literature mentions five different steps in raganuga bhakti. The *Vaishnava* poets have described these as five stages in the love of Radha and Krishna; but beware of supporting your weaknesses by this. It is impersonal, although the language is personal and romantic. In this literature the bhakta is considered to be a woman, and God a man. The language is figurative.

The first step is *purva raga.* This means "fundamental or primary attachment"; new love. The characteristics of purva raga are that you like to hear people speak appreciatively about your God. You listen with rapt attention. Also, you are effusive and enthusiastic in discussing Him. The attitude of rapt listening is called *sravana.* The spontaneous outflow of feelings when you talk about your Ideal is called *Kirtana.* (Group singing of bhaktas is also called kirtana.)

The second step is *kalaha,* which means the spirit of finding fault or quarrelling; but love is not lost. It is the beginning of the coming into prominence of the "I am" of the devotee. This expedites love and makes it more impetuous.

The next is *abhisara,* which means defiance for the sake of love. Defiance of custom, tradition or environment to show and to feel the strength of your love. (Here we find the spirit of "elopement.") And defiance grows with the seeking of advantage.

The next stage is *mana.* Here there is a feeling of pique, an assumed indifference, to arouse the intensity of love. The devotee neglects the object of his love. He wants to do without the Beloved because the Beloved has not shown any warmth of feeling. In a sense, he seeks to torture the object of love. But in his innermost heart he loves Him.

When we were children we sometimes showed pique at something that was said to us by our mother. We would say, "I won't eat!" And would go into our room and close the door. After a while, when we found mother unresponsive, we would softly open the door and hang a sign on it reading, "Ask me again." It is assumed anger.

It is self-importance which is behind mana. Love is something which is leading us to a higher goal. The elements have to be purified. Love does not gain force unless it goes through these stages of purification.

The next step is *viraha*, which means remaining in separation. It means the most intense state of longing. This makes love come to the boiling point; it sets in motion something which purifies the relationship even more. (Example: Krishna leaving Brindavan.)

These five steps of raganuga bhakti lead to *milana,* or union. The yearning of the devotee is fulfilled to a certain extent. It is the feeling of nearness to the Ishtam. Although it is lacking in completion, there is peace in the feeling of the nearness to one's Ishtam. It is the melting of the two, the *I* and the *Thou,* the *self* and the Ishtam. But, if there is union there must be eventual separation, so this state is defective. However, it is a peaceful state; the vessel is filled to the brim.

Through all these stages of raganuga bhakti the devotee has to keep his sraddha intact and unyielding. To meet the difficulties, the devotee should rather increase his sraddha. Sraddha is confidence in one's own self and in one's capacity and ability to overcome obstacles. It also means faith in the guru. If you have that sraddha, that faith and love, in spite of everything, in spite of all hardships, you will rise above suffering and enter into the state of prema. If faith is lost, everything is lost. It is a question of persistence. Slowly, steadily one should proceed; then one is sure of success.

Love is a God-given power, given to us without cost; and there is an abundant supply of it. But from it we create poison. Remember, whatever your environment, you can draw from that storehouse of infinite love. If you do not do so, you become bankrupt; you become a pauper for whom everything has dried up. Love, love in the midst of hell even! Create beauty in the midst of the ugly and the repulsive. Say, "Come what may— rain, storm, hail, snow—I am not going to swerve from my course of expressing that God-given power, love." Otherwise, a little headache, a little difficulty, a few obstacles, and you become discouraged; you cannot advance. That is idleness. That is laziness in love. Get rid of indolence. Meet all the obstructions that come—and then *ask for more!*

Before we discuss prema bhakti, let us pause to consider the practices already dealt with. By following even the first two practices of vaidhi bhakti, niyama and nishtha, and carrying them to the highest state, one can be led to perfection. When just beginning, we cannot expect each aspect of love to appear fully developed in our characters. In any case, human nature is so constituted that if a group of things is presented to it, it favours a particular one or two. The mind is so constituted. Even if a person cultivates all the six stages of practice in vaidhi bhakti he would lean more towards one or two than to the others. The personality of one person might be characterized by his excellence in dinata, another by seva or dhyana, and so on.

The question may be asked: does the devotee as he proceeds from one step to another transcend the previous discipline? When he reaches the raganuga state, does he do away with all those aspects we have considered under vaidhi bhakti? I do not say that he violates them; but there are a few practices in which he might slacken- and the emphasis on some might be different or might expand.

As your devotion grows your nishtha may become more subtle with less of a gross and more of a subtle tenacity. Puja may become more mental, and japam performed in a different way. Before, you might have been particular about the number of times you repeated the mantram, and you kept track of the count. Perhaps you repeated it 20,000 times a day. When japam becomes spontaneous, you do not keep track of the number. It goes on automatically, with your breathing. You perform your japam in many ways, in a temple or a shrine, in a school, a hospital, or any-where else. Then it is constant; you are hardly ever separated from it. Remembrance of your Ishtam, smaranam, flows naturally in your consciousness. Dhyana becomes deeper and the Ishtam, the Deity, is perceived in the lotus of your heart.

Dinata might be understood in a broader sense. When you grow to feel the existence of the inner Divinity you put yourself, your body, and your mind in the position of a servant of the Divinity, here, within you, and present everywhere. If a man begins to realize that his God is present everywhere, and he has the consciousness of being a servant of that God, he cannot but show real humility.

Seva becomes active service to God, with the attitude that all recipients are manifestations of God. Service to God in humanity is a great truth that will harmonize science and religion. As the bhakta progresses, seva is gradually established in every activity of his life.

Atmasamarpanam, or surrender to God, becomes more natural. Instead of consciously trying to hold on to the hand of God for fear of falling, we feel a great joy at His nearness and offer everything, joy and sorrow, at His blessed feet. We learn to feel that "He carries on his shoulders whatever the devotee needs" [Bhagavad-Gita]. We offer the practice and the results of the practice to God. We begin to feel the divine presence everywhere.

The disciplines and practices of bhakti yoga progress through these different stages, slowly and imperceptibly, until the character becomes pure and freed from selfishness and attachment. Although the practices of one stage may differ from those of another, one does not lose the benefits of the disciplines one has gone through. The preliminary disciplines of the first stage are added to one's character and become an integral part of it. In fact, these disciplines of yoga are the huge stones on which the foundations of great spiritual characters have been built. We admire great spiritual characters. We are often amazed and look upon them with wonder, but we are apt to forget that they were created by hard and sincere work, by persistence, by disciplines, and by hard practice. They have been through the "fire" test.

3

THERE is no lasting peace in either vaidhi or raganuga bhakti. So long as we hold on to the little self, we have to accept the sufferings, as well as the joys, of our devotion. They are the two sides of the same coin. It is our excessive ego-consciousness that is responsible for all our troubles on the path of bhakti. There are certain obstructions and dangers which are caused, in the main, by this faulty-ego-consciousness. We shall discuss these at this stage.

Emotion is like a living organism. If the proper direction for the different stages of its development is not supplied, it degenerates. Sometimes, even with proper direction, if love is not controlled it may degenerate. Bhakti cultivates undivided love—a passion, in fact—for God, the highest Ideal of the bhakta. It is heightened by rituals and other spiritual practices. If this great power of love is not well-controlled and balanced we can be harmed rather than helped by it. Furthermore, it is dangerous to direct this force only partially, not carrying it to its logical conclusion. One must proceed through the whole process of bhakti yoga, exercising control and maintaining balance. If this great force is not controlled, it may take a wrong channel and lead to many abnormalities.

Because of the inherent existence within us of absolute perfection, we are never satisfied. We are instinctively trying to find satisfaction in the outer world of the senses, the only world we know. This may take the form of the sex instinct. Fundamentally, of course, all instinct is a religious instinct. But the sex instinct is one of the greatest obstructions in the path of spiritual development, for it binds man to the world of the senses.

If real love for God is in the heart, it gives constructive direction to the emotional processes of the spiritual aspirant. But bhakti may degenerate into the worst form of material attachment and sensuality if the highest Ideal is not meditated upon regularly and carefully. One may become a slave to the senses. We must guard against the mundane life, against shifting the ideal. Through his practices, a bhakta's senses are heightened, and he is liable to become sensual. Never lose of the divine form of the Ishtam. The senses can never be satisfied; transcend their appeal. Contact the divine source within.

Bhakti may be heightened by mechanical means, such as music and rhythmic dancing. However, most of those who reach the state of ecstasy by such means cannot control themselves when the ecstasy is over. You all know of the sects here, in the West, such as the Holy Rollers who reach a pitch of religious fervour by rolling and jumping about. They come down from the height of their ecstasy as fast as they go up, like little rockets shot into the air.

There was a group of bhaktas in India who spent hours in singing religious songs and in other religious rituals and ceremonies and then robbed and murdered on their way home.* Abnor-

---

*Quite possibly the Swami's reference is to the infamous Thugs, a band of religious fanatics that worshipped the goddess Kali with offerings of murdered travellers. They were routed and ultimately stamped out by the British in the middle of the nineteenth century. [Ed.]

mal cruelty, criminality, and sensuality are found among so-called religious people; seldom among atheists.

If energy is held in a bottle, it is eager to express itself. Bhakti is the energy; our bodies and minds are the bottles. The energy within has to be controlled and properly directed to constructive channels of expression. The misapplication of that energy results in degeneration.

The remedy for sensuality is creative art 'and humanitarian service. Artistic expression is a great channel for the outflow of the feelings. Monks in medieval times used this channel for the expression of their emotions. Social work is also suitable as an outlet for some people.

In the development of the emotions, the intellectual and artistic faculties are kindled to a high degree. Learn control. Follow the steps outlined in bhakti yoga with regularity and care. Infinity contacting Infinity generates peace and contentment. The faculty of looking to the Divine within should be sharpened and kept shining.

We should not neglect the body, or engage in senseless austerity. The body is a machine; the only such machine we have to work with. Its value and proper place should be understood.

We must beware of mental reaction, when one expects too much too soon, when one exaggerates one's own importance. Such a bhakta is bound to run into disappointment. In reaction, he sometimes even develops strong hatred, jealousy, or anger—even towards his Ishtam. It has been said: "Though you feed a snake pure milk, it will still create poison."

It is not so difficult to gain ground as it is to hold it. It is gaining ground and then holding it that is essential. One must become "drunk" with love for God. But the process must be well-regulated. One must follow all the required steps carefully. An elephant enters a small pool of water; what havoc is created! We have to increase the capacity of the "pool" of our mind so that bhakti, even of the magnitude of an elephant, may enter it without throwing the pool into a tempest. The remedy for our reactions is constructive work, social and manual, and constant meditation upon the Ideal, following disciplines designed to subjugate the little ego, the cause of all the trouble.

Sri Ramakrishna told a wonderful story to illustrate degeneration in spiritual life. He said once that while he was going in a carriage to Fort William, in Calcutta, he did not realize until he reached his destination that he had been going down a gradually sloping road. (The fort is four stories below the surface.) It was not apparent that the carriage was going downhill. Degeneration in spiritual life is sometime so gradual that we do not realize we are on the downward path.

There are other impediments in bhakti, such as bigotry, fanaticism, mental slavery, and rank superstition. Zealots and the worst fanatics are produced by the misapplication of emotional energy. Some people swing to the extreme of fanaticism, thereby creating more noise in this already too noisy world! The remedy is to regulate emotion with reason and discrimination and to keep ourselves occupied.

Without reason and logic, religion can easily degenerate into the worst kind of superstition. Is religion such a falsehood that it cannot stand the light of day? There is nothing mysterious about religion or about bhakti. Such an attitude may easily develop into a slavery to dogmas and forms, without progressing in an understanding of the place of reason and logic in religious culture. You have a right to ask the "why" and "wherefore." One needs the stimulus of good company to prevent oneself from brooding and to keep the mind alert.

Swami Vivekananda once told a superstitious boy to forget religion for a while and go to a gymnasium and exercise his body. He added, "Kill an elephant and eat it!" Superstitious people often have weak bodies; a healthy body means a healthy mind.

Sanctimonious people are often superstitious. Swami Vivekananda once said that it would be better for some young men to play football instead of reading the Gita. He meant that they were weak, physically, mentally, and spiritually, and mere lip-service to the Gita meant nothing at all. Where was their *spiritual* strength?

Then there are the comparatively rare but very serious dangers in the path of bhakti, such as various obsessions, manias, fears and near madness. These are conditions which require expert attention, and each case has to be dealt with individually. Fortunately, these instances are rare.

There is another obstruction which may develop in the later stages of bhakti. After a devotee practises for some years, the obstruction of *satisfaction* may come. In Sanskrit this is called *tushti,* or the satisfaction of gaining some material, occult, intellectual, or spiritual powers. After undergoing many privations, a man may find that material things seem to come his way almost miraculously; or he sees occult manifestations that others do not see; or he may become an acknowledged intellectual, a leader or an authority, or may receive a little spiritual insight by his meditation. These are nothing but obstructions to his growth. The remedies are discrimination, good company, and the help of the guru.

In spite of the dangers and obstructions on the path of bhakti, it is a very natural way to reach perfection. By one-pointed devotion to the Ishtam, the aspirant may realize the highest goal; but sincerity, simplicity, and selfless devotion are required.

We now come to the third stage through which a bhakta must pass before he attains realization of his bhava. It is called prema bhakti. The discipline of bhakti yoga is an incessant process of making the proud and stubborn ego thinner until it is a mere "dot." That is prema.

The state of union in milana, the highest step in raganuga bhakti, is defective because where there is union there is also, eventually, separation. Love must reach the stage of highest purity or there can be no lasting peace in love. Purification of love is brought about by eliminating selfishness. In vaidhi and raganuga the "Thou" had to be sacrificed before the altar of "me" and "mine"; whereas, in prema, it is "Thou" and "Thou" *alone* which exists. There was a feeling of resentment in the raganuga state because God did not answer our call; yet there was enjoyment in hearing our own voice calling, "God! God!"

When the turbulence of raganuga has subsided, prema appears. It is the state of "not I, but Thou"; of pure, uncaused love, love which makes no demands, which gives and wants nothing in return. It is love that seeks no gratification. In that state love flows from the devotee into the object of adoration with no ulterior motive. Pure love flows without cause. Because a thing is beautiful I love that thing—that is caused love. Love that has been caused owing to the presence of some quality or characteristic in the object of love cannot last. It is subject to change, dimunition, degeneration.

We have to develop uncaused love. Our love should be so perfect that it flows without reason; that it remains unchanged in all circumstances; that it always gives and never seeks to take.

Until we have attained to that stage, our love is not real love.

Prema comes after we have passed through the other two stages. It is the pure "gold" from which all impurities have been eradicated during the earlier two stages. This is the stage of prema. There is not the slightest intention of receiving anything in return for your love. In prema, love is freed from the dross of "I". The merging of the "I" into the "Thou" is complete. And when the "I" is relinquished, union between the devotee and his Ishtam takes place.

A Persian poet tells the story of the lover who came to the door of his beloved. In answer to his knock, she called out "Who is there?"

"It is I," came the voice from outside. The door did not open.

Again he knocked. "Who is there?" she asked.

"I am, thy beloved," answered the lover. Still the door remained closed.

The persistent lover knocked a third time. This time, in answer to her query he called out, completely forgetting himself, "It is thyself, Beloved!" And the door was opened. That is the attitude of prema.

Sri Ramakrishna tells the story of the cow who always says: "*Hamba! Hamba!*" ("I! I!") and so has to suffer many indignities. It has to plough the fields day in and day out. When it is old it may be dragged to the slaughter house and killed. Its hide is stretched and made into a drum and is beaten hard and mercilessly. Some of it is made into shoes and ground into the dust of the streets. It is only when its entrails are tautly stretched on the carder's bow that it finally cries out, "*Tuhu! Tuhu!*" ("Thou! Thou!"). Only after so much misery with its "Hamba! Hamba!" can the cow finally reach the state where it says, "Tuhu."

The characteristics of prema bhakti are:

1. Complete surrender of the ego to the object of love, with no demands; renunciation of the little self; and no desire for gratification of the senses.

2. Prema is subjective. The bhakta feels happiness within, not outside himself. There is no suffering in this kind of love. The mind that always finds the cause of everything outside itself, believing, for instance, that enjoyment comes from the flower, that joy and suffering are caused by something or someone outside itself,

lives in a state of "objectivity." The mind which finds the cause, the source, of everything *within* has the "subjective" attitude. That man can say: "I love my own soul. I love the contact with my God within. And I can declare that I do not love with the expectation that my love will be returned. I love because I *love* to love!"

Love, in the last analysis, is the search for one's bigger, more mighty, more perfect Self. I see my Self reflected in you, and I think it is you I love. That is our condition.

The object which you think you love is only your own face in the mirror, which reflects your mood or ideal. It is the face of your real Self.

You do not love a thing or a person if there is no reflection of your Self in it. Why does the artist love his violin? He finds that ideal of beauty he has cherished in his heart when he plays on his violin. His own inner ideal finds expression through the instrument.

But the "song of love" always remains within. It will never be sung to the satisfaction of any singer or listener. Love is God, love is infinite. We can never bring it down to the level of the finite.

3. Prema is idealistic. In this state the bhakta's life becomes just a tenure of loving service. There is no competition or contest in the spirit of service to his beloved God. The bhakta feels supreme authority in his relationship with God, yet he is extremely humble and modest. He enjoys satisfaction in that love; he lives for that supreme love, which he carefully nurtures in his heart. This gives beauty to every contact in his life. He enjoys the love subjectively; he covers everything with it. There is always a feeling of lack of attainment which makes for continuous progress. In prema, love is not dependent upon any condition time, or place. The bhakta enjoys happiness in spite of everything.

4. In the state of prema, love becomes universal. The bhakta recognizes his beloved God everywhere, in everything. When your spiritual practices bear their finest fruit the God who was a presence to you, composed of form, melts away in the melting pot of your love, and conceals Himself in everything. The beloved God is recognized in everything and in every place. You are thus in touch with Him every moment of your life. In the state of prema the object of love is projected into everything in the universe. One becomes a *vishwa-premi,* a lover of the universe. The

highest state of prema bhakti is abstract.

Merging oneself into the Ishtam, which is the highest state of bhakti yoga, is called bhava samadhi. Bhava samadhi is the fulfilment, the revelation, of any one of the bhavas. The Ishtam becomes alive and real, even in the case of a statue or a picture. It is the physical reality of the Ishtam. When the bhakta reaches this exalted state, his bhava expands from a limited to a universal aspect, from the specific to the formless.

For instance, in santa bhava the bhakta finds the God of his adoration as the universal Spirit, present in all things. Everything reflects his Ishtam. He sees Him behind all the masks of human faces. Sri Ramakrishna realized God through this bhava, as well as through others. For some time he could not pluck flowers, for he saw the divine Spirit in them. He felt God in a blade of grass and could not bear for the grass to be walked upon. He said that everything was filled with the divine Spirit, as pillows are stuffed with the same thing, though they appear outwardly different. This is a peaceful and calm recognition of God in all things.

The attitude of the dasya bhava, of service to a beloved master, grows from the specific to the formless. The Ishtam, the Master of the devotee, first appears in a form and then it expands and expands until it reaches infinity. The form vanishes and becomes the All.

Tata bhava, or the attitude of a child toward its parent, also develops from the specific to the formless. Jesus's devotion to his Father and the devotion of Sri Ramakrishna for the Mother are two glowing examples of the highest attainment through this bhava. Ramakrishna saw the Mother in a form and also saw Her everywhere. Even in some of the lowest types of persons, he saw only his beloved Mother. His devotion to the Mother and his realization of unity behind all the world's seeming diversity is one of the greatest revelations of universal truth ever put before humanity.

The devotee following the sakhya bhava finds his beloved God, his Friend, everywhere.

In vatsalya bhava, the devotee has the attitude of being not only the father or mother of his Ishtam, but of the whole world. He looks upon all people as his own children. From being the mother of the Ishtam, one grows to become the universal Mother, seeing the beloved Child everywhere.

The bhakta who has followed the madhura bhava finds his

Beloved present always. The Beloved has "hidden" Himself within all persons and things in the universe. Thus the bhakta is never separated from Him.

Those who have attained to the exalted state of bhava samadhi have all realized the same thing, though their attitudes are different. In all the bhavas the Ishtam becomes universal. Subjectively, the realizations are the same. However, according to their external, objective manifestations these great souls may be classified under the following headings:

1. *Jada*—statue-like, sunk in meditation, oblivious of everything. He may sit without moving for years. He is waited upon and fed by others. Otherwise, his body would cease to live, and would "fall off."

2. *Bala*—childlike, like a child of five years, with such a childlike simplicity in his external expression. (Sri Ramakrishna is an example of this bhava samadhi.)

3. *Unmatta*—crazy or drunken. He acts like an intoxicated man; for he is drunk with the wine of divine love.

4. *Pisacha*—horrible to look at, frightening. This attitude may come because he prefers to be left alone and unmolested.

5. *Raja-rajeswara*—like the king of all kings. He carries himself like a great king. Abundance follows him wherever he goes.

Although these five types are widely different, we should remember that all of them have attained the same goal. We only classify them according to their outward appearances. All have the same realization; the inner consciousness is the same. The explanation for the fact that these realized souls remain in such vastly different states is that it is due to their *prarabdha karma*. Prarabdha karma is unchangeable karma, the results of actions in previous lives. This karma must exhaust itself. This is so, even in the lives of those who have realized the goal of spiritual life.

The state of pisacha may be the most difficult for us to understand. It may be illustrated by a beautiful happening which occurred at the Dakshineswar temple, shortly after it was dedicated.

One day a "madman" walked into the temple grounds. He was dressed in the rags of a beggar, dirty and unkempt. He carried in one hand a twig from a tree and in the other a potted plant. He was so mad-looking that even the beggars shunned him. When it was time to eat the food from the temple offerings, the beggars would not allow him to sit with them. So he walked over to a rubbish heap and began to eat the garbage along with the stray dogs who had gathered there. He threw one arm over the back of one of the dogs. Sometimes he would give a dog a push, so he could reach the food. The dogs did not seem to mind. Together they ate in peace.

Sri Ramakrishna's cousin, Haladhari, was in the shrine at that time and he saw all of this. He ran to Ramakrishna and told him about the man, and together they went to talk to him. The "madman" spoke the highest wisdom to them, but to others he would say nothing. Later, as he was leaving the temple grounds, Hriday, Ramakrishna's nephew, ran after him, begging for some instruction. The man at first paid no heed to him, but when Hriday implored him, the man turned around and said: "When the filthy water in this ditch and the water of the sacred Ganges appear the same to you, then know you have realized the goal." And he disappeared down the road. Ramakrishna said that the man was a *paramahamsa*.

Those who have realized the highest are called paramahamsas. Literally, the word means "great goose." The simile comes from an old story that there exists a species of geese which can draw out only the milk from a mixture of milk and water; that is, separate the real from the unreal or non-essential. If one wants to plant rice one must be interested in both the husk and the grain. But to one who wants to eat rice the husk is not necessary. It is non-essential and one dispenses with it. One who has been able to discover Divinity, the Real, behind every manifestation is a paramahamsa.

All systems of religion and philosophy have tried to remove the mystery of death, have tried to peep into the future. Life-after-death existence according to bhakti yoga has been dealt with in Chapter VI of the Bhagavad-Gita.

On no account does a bhakta want to be one with God. He wants to love God. He sees beauty in everything, in the external as well as the internal world. He says: "I do not want to *be* sugar; I want to *eat* sugar." The bhakta hates the word, *mukti*, or freedom. He does not consider himself bound, so he avoids such words as freedom and liberation. The bhakta does not appreciate losing his identity, even in God.

The primary goal of the bhakta is to cultivate and emulate God within himself. He finds no superfluity in mankind; he sees

Y—11

beauty in everything. His inner world is the source of all beauty. He always remembers that his heart is the parlour of God.

The bhakta says, "My world is not maya, but a playground. What difference if I am reincarnated with wings or with a tail and horns? I love variety. I want to come again to enjoy my bhakti. It is fun! If my Beloved wants to play, why, so must I!"

Regarding after-death existence, a bhakta wants to go to a region which will give him the fulfilmnt of all his devotional desires, without any of the shortcomings of the material earthworld. Such a region, which is more than the conception of a heaven, is called *Vaikuntha* (without defect or imperfection). Vaikuntha is a plane of existence made of *chinmaya*. Objects there are seen as in a dream. There the bhakta attains the body he desires, a body composed of bliss minus the shortcomings of the flesh; a body capable of rendering unlimited service to his God. This body is immune from disease and decomposition. The bhakta wishes to enjoy forever, without any interruption, the divine revelation. In Vaikuntha all devotional desires are totally fulfilled. The bhakta is never separated from his Ishtam. His contact with his God is tangible, natural, and normal. Such a contact, such a state, the bhakta believes to be eternal. The bhakta wants to adore his Ishtam for ever. Even though he may see his Ishtam everywhere, it still remains the object of his devotion. He does not want to be one with God; he wants only to *love* God.

According to the literature of bhakti yoga, there are four relationships a bhakta may enjoy in Vaikuntha:

1. *Sarupya*—meaning "with the same or equal form, sameness of form with the Ishtam." Here on earth the bhakta meditates on the form of the Ishtam. The meditation on that form will give him the same chinmaya form.

2. *Sayujya*—constantly attached to, or with, the Ishtam. A union with the Ishtam in which any relationship may be enjoyed.

3. *Salokya*—belonging to the same sphere or region. In any form, but in the same region. (It is like being able to visit the President at the White House, but not remaining there always.) You are not constantly with the Ishtam, but you are on the same plane of existence.

4. *Sarshti*—with equal power or rank. The reflection of the power of the Ishtam, of God, is upon you. You have all the power of God, except the power of creation.

In life or in death, or in whatever existence he finds himself, the bhakta's sole interest is to love his beloved God. The great bhaktas of the world, the great mystics, have lived intensely emotional lives, but they are great because that emotion was balanced by their devotion to their Ideal.

The love of God is inexhaustible.

Let your attitude be that every act is an offering of devotion. Find God, and be concerned with Him alone.

IV

KARMA YOGA
The Path of Selfless Work

I

Man is potentially divine. His perfection is disturbed by agitations caused by his setting into motion the wheel of causation. This results in action and reaction, which produces karma. Until karma is effaced, man cannot be perfect or express his inner perfection. He cannot be free.

THIS is the theory, proposition, and goal of karma yoga. Karma yoga is the method of attaining perfection through action or work. Action is inherent in the nature of all living creatures. It cannot be avoided. Since it cannot be avoided, this inevitable factor of life can be utilized, through following the path of karma yoga, as a means of reach perfection, to express potential perfection.

The impulse for expression, the struggle against obstacles that stand in the way of the expression of our inner divinity, is life. No living organism in this world can remain without activity even for a single moment. God Himself is working incessantly. If there is any entity that cannot look forward to a vacation, it is poor God! He must be working every moment. Otherwise, the whole of creation would fall into chaos. It is God's activity that holds this universe together, just as a thread holds the jewels of a beautiful necklace together and in place. Through every activity is woven God's activity. Through His incessant work, which finds expression everywhere, this whole universe is kept in a wonderful order of love, beauty, and utility.

The sun, the moon, the stars, the planets, our earth with all its mountains, oceans, seas, rivers, plains, trees and flowers, beasts and birds—in fact, every atom in the universe—are all constantly active. Nothing can remain inactive for a single moment.

Our nature is constantly urging us to expand ourselves and

to attain the state of perfection. It is this which compels us to go out into the field of action. So there can never be any question as to whether we should work or not, because it is our very nature that will send us out, in spite of our resistance, into the field of action.

The question is this: how can we work so that whatever we do brings the realization of that perfection within us? The urge for expression is a mighty force. If we follow it blindly it leads us into many difficulties. Desire is never satisfied. The more we get the more we want; it goes on and on. This urge must be controlled and regulated. Hindu philosophy teaches that this basic urge for expression can be converted into a method for attaining spiritual illumination.

How can we be spiritual in the street as well as in retreat? Are we to be saints on Sundays and sinners on weekdays? In other words, is our daily life at war with our spiritual progress? If you are seeking a philosophy of life by which you may harmonize activity with spirituality. you will have to dig into Sanskrit literature to find it.   I make bold to say that nowhere else in the world will you find that golden bridge except there.   India lives in order to give this message to the world.   Believe me if you will, or call me crazy if you wish, but the fact is this: it is the philosophy of India, especially her philosophy of karma, or work, that is going to be the future religion of the world.

The word karma is derived from the Sanskrit root *kri*, "to do". It literally means everything we do—all our actions, both physical and mental.   Let us take a grammatical simile: every verb you use after the pronoun "I" is karmic.   I see, I hear, I want, I think— the "I" is the subject of all these actions.   The verb denotes action (and implies a reaction).   Technically, the word karma also means the subtle law of cause and effect, in which the results of one's actions form the cause of future events.   Anything that sets in motion a force of causation is karma.

Yoga means to yoke or join together. In the sense it is used here it means to "join" the lower self of man to the higher Self, or perfection, which is our real nature. Karma yoga, therefore, means the path of attainment to this union through karma or action.   It is fully an independent method as good as devotion, meditation, or discrimination for the realization of the divine perfection inherent in man.

By following the path of karma yoga, we learn the secret of how to utilize our daily actions to achieve this great end. We learn how to cut the thread of cause and effect that binds us to the lower self. As long as the force of causation remains active in a human being, he is not perfect, he is not free. Freedom, for a karma yogin (a follower of this path) lies in the total destruction, or neutralization, of his karma. The force of causation has two aspects: the link of causation and its expression. The yogi wants to cut the link of causation to free himself from the yoke of karma and its effects. He also wants to express himself in such a way that his work will cause no disturbance to his mind. The subjective aspect of karma yoga is the endeavour to cut short the chain of causation and be free. A karma yogin endeavours to rise above the law of cause and effect. The right subjective attitude leads him to transcend this law.

Man must work in the objective field of action in such a way that he will manifest, more and more, his inner perfection through his work. At the same time, the subjective attitude towards his work must be such that the work does not bind him, but contributes to his inner development. So, you see, there are two aspects to karma yoga, the subjective and the objective.

Perfection is within. Desire creates disturbances in our consciousness which keep that perfection from manifesting itself. Activity with desire leads to the greed of possession which forges the chain of attachment to "I and mine." Nothing belongs to anyone. Never seek to establish ownership of anyone or anything. Do not even say, "*My* body". Say, "*The* body". There are several attitudes one may adopt in order to overcome this idea of possession.

Desire and attachment, the inseparable twins, create the relationship of cause and effect. The chain of cause and effect leads the soul to births and deaths and keeps it limited. Mental karma is even more serious than physical karma because it affects consciousness more deeply. The obstruction, then, is that of desire and attachment. Karma yoga teaches us how to control these. Action with desire, whether physical or mental, creates karma which must exhaust itself by its effects. When the effects are exhausted, man is free. The attempt of the karma yogin is to accelerate this process.

Karma, or actions, may be considered from several aspects.

For instance, our thoughts and actions may be classified under two general headings: Action for the achievement of desired ends and the attainment of wishes (*ishta-prapti*); action in order to avoid undesired issues (*anishta-parihara*), or action done in fear of achieving undesired ends. Regarding man, there is another type of karma called "compensatory karma" which apparently overlaps the previous two classifications, but which is occasional and unavoidable. The endeavour to compensate bad action by good, such as an apology or the making of amends for some previous action, is compensatory karma. Confession in the Catholic Church might be considered under this heading.

From the point of view of results, karma may be classified in several ways: (1) karma that brings the result of desirable ends; (2) karma that brings the result of undesired ends, or unhappiness and suffering; and (3) karma that is neutral. Our effort in karma yoga is to reduce our actions to this third type of karma. The chain of good and bad action must be neutralized.

There is another type of karma called "involuntary karma", wherein self-consciousness is not involved. This kind of karma does not create any results. But is there really such a thing as involuntary karma? Raja yoga teaches that such involuntary action as the beating of one's heart can be consciously controlled. If this is so, then that action, seemingly involuntary, is merely a dormant voluntary action. But conscious action always sets in motion a "wave," good or bad, within the consciousness that creates karma.

Karma, again, may be classified as action that is good and constructive or bad and destructive. What is the criterion of good or bad action? An action is good if it uplifts the doer and produces the greatest amount of happiness for the greatest number of people. The reverse of this is considered bad. Essentially, to be good, any action has to uplift the agent. A good action helps you unfold your inner divinity. If, by thought or deed, you put a wall of narrowness around yourself, keeping aloof and separate from the rest of the world, you deny your divine Self, no matter what that action is. I call such action destructive and unspiritual. From the spiritual standpoint, our action is good only when it helps to remove the barrier of egoism and expand the soul, thereby helping us to realize, more and more, that fundamental unity. that Oneness which is behind the universe.

Generally speaking, an action is considered good if it conforms to certain relative conceptions of right and wrong, good and bad. But an action which is good under some circumstances may be bad in others. There are four tests of good or right actions: (1) a good action must conform to the fundamental conception of truth; (2) it should not go against religious or temporal laws; (3) it should conform to the unwritten customs and traditions observed by good people of the particular society in which one happens to live; (4) good action should bring satisfaction, never a feeling of regret. But the absolute standard for good or bad action is: *That which does not veil or contradict the recognition of the basic truth of Oneness in everything is good action; that which obscures this truth is bad.*

To attain the highest freedom through karma yoga you have to free yourself *within* from the bondage even of good action. But you have to take advantage of good action in order to check the current of bad or destructive activity. Sri Ramakrishna used to say that if you get a thorn in your foot while walking in the woods you take another thorn to remove it. Then you throw both thorns away. A good action rids you of a bad action. But the aim is to rise above both, to *free yourself within* from the bondage of all action.

No living organism can remain stationary; life itself is constant activity. There is no rest except in the Infinite. "Then why do anything at all?" you may ask. "Why should we not all be lazy, and do nothing?" So long as the influence of maya hangs over us, so long as we belong to the gigantic wheel of life, there is no option for us to do or not to do. Do, we must! It is the revolving of that big wheel that thrusts us into the field of action in spite of our resistance.

Every action is the result of previous action; it is also the cause of subsequent actions. The chain is threefold: cause—karma, effect. Effect again becomes the cause of further karma, and on and on it goes. The question, "Who set the wheel of karma in motion?" is like asking which came first, night or day, the hen or the egg. If we enter a room and a wheel is revolving so rapidly that it obscures a light which is behind it, does knowing who set the wheel in motion help us to see the light? No. *The wheel must be stopped.*

Let us analyze karma from the viewpoint of the law of causation.

1. *Sanchita karma*—stored-up, accumulated karma. It is like a jar of seeds ready to be planted. Nothing happens without a cause. An accumulated force of causation is utilized in different ways. Unused potentiality may be drawn upon at will. This explains a suddenly acquired ability.

2. *Kriyamana karma*—progressive, continuous karma. The field of our existence is now being occupied by this karma. It is that part of causation which is now working on the surface, evidently and palpably, producing its results. It is that karma which we recognize right now, of which we can trace the cause.

3. *Prarabdha karma*—karma that is discharged and is unalterable from the standpoint of our present knowledge. There are two kinds of energy, potential and released. Prarabdha karma is released karma or energy. It is the force which has, therefore, gone out of control. Prarabdha karma has determined our present life as regards sex, parentage, special abilities, tendencies, talents, and the environment of our birth. Therefore, certain endeavours in life covered by prarabdha karma cannot be altered by us. Lest it encourage indolence, we should ignore it. Although it may sometimes create a disadvantage, prarabdha karma does not stand in the way of attaining perfection. Suppose a man is born with some physical deformities. He may not be able to alter such defects but they will not interfere with his attaining perfection in his spiritual life. This type of karma reminds us we should accept facts as facts. Do not exaggerate hopes and aspirations. Do not strive after the impossible.

We are accountable for every detail of our lives through a specific urge or impetus. Knowledge is not conclusive proof of what we are. Memory is no evidence. Action always produces action. A specific karma gives you a particular incarnation whereby you work in a certain field of endeavour, at the same time creating numerous subsidiary karmas. We are born with a burden of karma and whether we like it or not, that burden has to be worked out.

The three types of karma mentioned have been beautifully illustrated in a classic simile. An archer has a stock of arrows in a quiver on his back. They represent sanchita karma. He has an arrow in his hand ready to be discharged. It represents kriyamana karma. The arrow which he has already discharged, and which is speeding on its way to the target, represents prarabdha karma. Over this arrow he has no control. It must take its course.

In regard to sanchita and kriyamana karma, man can express freedom. Like the arrows in the archer's hand and in the quiver at his back, they are under control so long as the archer does not shoot them. Education, culture, and discipline control the way in which these may be used up or thrown aside altogether.

So far as prarabdha karma is concerned, the consequences, good or bad, have to be endured with patience until the effects are exhausted. If you disassociate yourself from the sanchita and kriyamana karma, there will be no karmic momentum left, other than the prarabdha, which will run its course without creating any more karmic complications. The karma yogin works out his prarabdha karma in such a way that it does not create any more karma to bind him. He controls kriyamana karma by discrimination. The sanchita, the stored-up tendencies, the potential action resulting from previous karma, he controls by proper analysis understanding, culture, and discipline.

A karma yogin wants to burn the force of causation of these three types of karma. A karma cannot be extinguished by avoidance or by neglecting the outer action. The *force* of it must be burnt away; the *seed* of its causation destroyed. Sri Ramakrishna supports this with these illustrations:

The fertility in grain is destroyed by frying it. So, karma can be "fried" and enjoyed and yet not produce any harvest. We must know the art of "frying" our karma!

A burnt rope has no power to bind. The burnt rope lies on the ground in the same shape as before it was burnt. It looks like a rope, but blow on it and it will vanish. We have to learn the secret of burning the "rope" of karma, thus making our actions powerless to bind us.

A steel sword that has touched the philosopher's stone turns into gold. It can no longer be used for destruction. A sword that has been turned into gold is kept only as a souvenir. Let every action be like a beautiful souvenir, like a sword that has been transformed and thereby lost its sharpness and power to hurt or kill any being.

When we learn the secret of karma yoga, life's actions have no power to bind us.

The law of karma differs from predestination in that since you have the power to release a force of causation you also have the power to check or undo it.

The difference between a karmi, a good worker, and a karma

yogin is that the work of the former is efficient, but does not lead to liberation. The difference lies in the attitude towards the work.

Consider your work as an exercise for the cultivation of the right attitude. This attitude may be: (1) To consider yourself as the witness of the action. Have no desire, nothing to attain by work. Work only because the lower self has to be "tired out" before it can attain eternal rest.

(2) To consider that it is God whom you are contacting in all relationships and in all work. Do your work as worship and service to God.

(3) To "work for the sake of work." To enjoy "intense rest in the midst of intense action" (Bhagavad-Gita).

The subjective attitude is assured if you maintain any of these attitudes towards your work. Your work then (a) becomes a means of reaching freedom; (b) becomes a form of worship, the highest form of worship; or, (c) becomes selfless work, work for the sake of work, which cannot bind you to the cycle of causation. A karma yogin throws self overboard and does his work without attachment, without desire for reward or results.

Stay absolutely aloof from the results of activity.

Do not register the acceptance of praise; digest it. Good or bad, pleasant or unpleasant, accept both sides of the coin. Then it doesn't matter if one throws a garland at you or an old pair of shoes!

Our nature is such that our work always takes a long stride ahead of us. Let the mind rest on the work. Do not think ahead to its future merit or demerit. In that way the mind will not become scattered in threads of hope, expectation, or anxiety. Always maintain mental repose. Let your consciousness be absorbed in the work or the undertaking at hand. In the process of inevitable activities, cultivate these attitudes.

The subjective aspect is the most important consideration in any action. Extreme sincerity is necessary. We become great by taking cognizance of our failures, not by supporting or whitewashing them.

Always act with the intention of giving instead of receiving. Then you will have the right subjective attitude. But in giving, do not become arrogant, desiring honour, and look not down upon the recipient. Do not think you are doing good to the world by your good actions. The world can get along very well without you! It is *you* who benefit by your good actions. Never think in terms of charity.

Giving is service to God. Not arrogant charity, but service. Life attains greatness, life attains power, life attains fulfilment, when we attain efficiency in this function of giving. Life should be lived with the intention of giving.

The hand that stretches like this, palm upwards, says, "I want something. Give me!" Always extend your hand palm downward, as in the act of giving.

I once knew a man who was very stingy by nature. Every day an acquaintance of his would give him something and then say to him, "Give that back to me."

When the man asked him why he gave things to him and then immediately asked him to return them, the other man replied, "I am just stretching your hand to teach you to give!"

A child who has the habit of stealing should be sent on errands of giving; then he will gradually be cured.

Give everything you have. You will be giving to God. It may sound difficult, but we are talking about something very high.

When your work is done in the spirit of service, service to a higher power, to God, or whatever your ideal may be, that karma is no karma. It is seva, service or worship of God. It does not bind one to the wheel of causation.

In the last analysis, there is only the subjective standard of action. Let your work be an exercise to enable you to feel that you are gaining inner strength. Realize that your real Self remains aloof and free from all activity.

The Gopi maidens were once making their way to a temple with their offerings of food. They came to a wide river. There was no way they could cross. Nearby they saw the hut of a holy man. They went to him seeking some assistance. The holy man said that first they should give him whatever food they had with them. They gave him their offerings. He ate everything there was to be eaten. He then walked to the edge of the river and said, "If there be truth in what I say, if I have not eaten anything, let this river part for the crossing of these maidens."

The little maidens were standing behind the old sage. When they heard this they were surprised. But the river parted and the little girls walked safely across to the other side. The sage knew that his "I" was above all the activity of his senses and body. He knew he was he Witness of the activity.

The slogan of karma yoga as laid down by Swami Vivekananda is: "Throw the self overboard; do whatever comes your way, and be free."

Once there was a thug who had lived all his life through robbery and hold-ups. His conscience was as wide as the gate to hell! He never stopped to think, about, much less hesitate to do, even the vilest of acts. However, he was passionately fond of his wife and children. That was the one good aspect of his otherwise terrible life. But that was not long granted to him, for in one sad disaster he lost his wife and all is children. He was left alone with the scar of cruelty as his sole companion.

This sudden shock, however served a purpose. It made him look within. But there he could see nothing but darkness covering darkness. He began to feel the pangs of remorse. As his mind began to dwell on his past misdeeds, he counted fifty-two murders written on the tablet of his memory! Ah! It is too much! How could he save himself from such a heavy burden of sin? He thought he would try to find some holy man and unburden himself to him.

After wandering about for some time, he came upon the retreat of a sage. The thug opened his conscience to the holy man, who advised him to stay in the retreat and render service to other holy men living there. He began to feel better in the holy company; but he did not dare to believe that his sins had left him. He had strong faith in the holy man, whose love for him he could never doubt, but he was anxious to have his sins expiated. He asked the holy man if he could undertake a pilgrimage to visit the holy shrines and bathe in the holy waters, with the hope of washing away his sins.

The holy man readily extended him permission and gave him a small black flag to take with him on his journey.

"Take this, my son," said the holy man. "This flag holds the marks of your sins. When it turns white, know that all your sins have been washed away. May you return to us, my son, with your conscience as white as snow."

There was not a holy shrine where the thug did not worship; there was no holy water in the whole country in which he failed to bathe. After the performance of each holy rite, he would quickly open his knapsack and take out the little flag to see if it had turned white. To his disappointment, he found that the flag remained as black as ever.

Knowing no more holy places to go to or any other expiatory rite to perform, he at last decided to go back to the hermitage of his master and render service to him, in humble submission, bearing the burden of his hopelessly irredeemable sins.

So he trudged back; through cities and through forests, towards the hermitage. One day after sunset he reached a place a few miles from the hermitage. He thought it would be better to spend the night there in the forest and proceed to the hermitage early next morning. He did not want to disturb the Brotherhood by arriving late at night. All around him there was deep calm. The only sound he heard was that of the crickets. Never before did nature appear so beautiful to him. There was beauty everywhere in that solemn darkness, everywhere except in the ugly face of the darkness within his heart. Tears rolled down his cheeks.

Suddenly the silence was broken by a human voice, the cry of a woman in distress. He jumped up and ran quickly in the direction of the cry. With the trained, catlike steps of a thug, he followed the direction of the sound and came upon a little clearing. What he saw there threw his blood into a tempest! Three ruffians were tormenting a helpless woman. He said to himself, "Do I dare attack these three men alone? If I manage to disable or even kill one of them, the others might be put to flight. Even if the remaining two attack me, can I not call upon my bygone skills and fight two men?"

Then another thought passed through his mind. "Suppose I can rescue this poor, helpless woman by killing one, two, or even all three of these men. The woman would be saved, no doubt. But what about me? Oh, soul of mine, can you bear a little more, just a little more than the already heavy burden of fifty-two murders?"

There was no time to lose. "Fifty-two or fifty-three, what does it matter?" he cried out, "My poor soul, to hell you will have to go! I save the girl at any cost!"

No sooner had he thrown his "self" overboard by this decision than he felt within him the strength of twenty lions. With a roar he dealt a mortal below to one of the ruffians; the others were put to flight. He picked up the poor woman, who collapsed in his arms.

The following morning he led the trembling girl towards the hermitage of the holy man. They were received by the Brotherhood, who, though surprised, asked no questions. They made the girl comfortable and asked their brother to rest for a while before seeing the holy man.

Later, he sat at the feet of the master, and related in detail the story of his adventure of the previous night. Everyone noticed that he looked pure and free. When he was asked about his pilgrimage and the little flag, he said, "Oh, I needn't bother any more about that foolish business." Then he turned to the master and said, "Master, take back your little black flag, which has turned even blacker. I don't care. I remain here for the rest of my life at your service."

He reached in his knapsack for the little flag. Instead of the black flag, there was one as white as snow! He looked at it with unchanged expression and said, "Master, black or white, I lay it at your feet. I am through with it. I have thrown self overboard. I don't want to know what will happen to me, so long as I can serve you."

The holy man said, "How can one avoid the consequences of evil deeds, when one still wants the fruit of one's meritorious deeds? They are like two sides of the same coin. Accept the one and you have to accept the other. The flag did not and could not lose a bit of its blackness so long as you were covetously eager to reap the fruit of your good actions. This is the reason why your pilgrimage and all the holy ceremonies could not remove the blackness from your conscience, although they accumulated some good karma. When, through the grace of the Lord, you could learn to consciously and deliberately reject the thought of all good or bad consequences, you transcended the law of karma, and became really free."

"Purity and freedom, my son," said the master, "are nothing but selflessness. Selflessness is fearlessness. Fearlessness is sinlessness."

2

KARMA YOGA does not interfere in any way with your objective expressions. Rather, it helps you to express yourself more skilfully and systematically. If you adopt the method of karma yoga and then follow your occupation, say, of a street cleaner, you will be the best street cleaner in the world. Moreover, you will be the highest of yogis. This method of karma yoga produces the fullest excellence in the objective as well as the subjective side of life. Furthermore, by following the method of karma yoga you may utilize your everyday occupation of making a living to attain spiritual perfection. A friend of mine* once said to me, "Making a living is too often just 'making a living', with no deeper significance." However, we can spiritualize "making a living". By being a butcher all your life you can become a Godman—through the method of karma yoga. Let me tell you a story.

There was a yogi who had practised hard disciplines for years—postures, breathing exercises, and so on. One day he was sitting under a tree in a forest when a little bird dropped some dirt on him. The yogi looked up in anger. His anger had such power that the little bird immediately fell to the ground, burnt to ashes. The yogi felt rather proud of this confirmation of his progress after all his years of practice.

Later that day he went to the nearby village, where he approached a house for alms. A woman's voice came from within, and asked him to wait a few minutes as she was busy serving her family. The yogi became irritated at this, having just that day seen what great powers he had! He called out again, this time rather sharply. The woman's voice again floated out to him from inside the house, "Have a little patience, yogi. Don't think that I am a little bird, that you can burn me!"

This remark amazed the yogi. When the woman finally came to the door, he asked her how she knew about the bird episode. She told him that she too followed a certain path of yoga. When he questioned her further, she replied, "Go on into the village and see the butcher. He will be able to explain everything to you."

"The butcher!" gasped the yogi.

The woman answered simply, "Yes, the butcher."

"What can a butcher teach me about yoga?" the yogi wondered. His curiosity was aroused, so he went to the village. From a distance he saw the butcher doing his butchering. The yogi was disgusted at the sight, and he felt like turning back and giving

---

*The Bengali writer, Dhan Gopal Mukherji.

up the whole unpleasant affair. However, he approached the shop. The butcher looked up from his work. "Oh, she has sent you," said the butcher, without waiting for the yogi to speak. "Would you mind waiting until I finish my work? Then I shall be glad to talk with you."

By this time the yogi's curiosity was thoroughly aroused. When the butcher had finished, he asked the yogi to accompany him to his home. There he excused himself again while he attended to his aged parents, bathed them, fed them, and made them comfortable.

At last, when he had finished all his duties, the butcher sat down and explained to the amazed yogi the method of attaining spiritual perfection through work, *any* work. This is the path of karma yoga.

Spirituality should not be considered an ephemeral or "other worldly" attainment. It should be regarded in terms of the skilfulness, the degree of perfection we are able to manifest in and through every one of our actions, even the most insignificant, and the attitude we have towards these actions. To be spiritual you do not have to sit in certain postures and breathe in specific ways. You do not have to be a recluse. You can practise your spiritual exercises anywhere, under any conditions and in every situation. The secret is to have the right attitude.

No matter what you are doing, see that you put yourself into it entirely. That is what I call real efficiency. Treat your work as an object of worship, or nearly so. Of course, I know that the word "worship" does not mean much nowadays. So, shall I say instead: *concentrate your whole energy on the work*. Know that through your work you are going to attain the highest spiritual perfection. Let nothing else exist for you. When work is done without desire, without attachment to results, with the attitude of manifesting the highest perfection through it, it is bound to be done skilfully and efficiently. Such work creates no disturbance in the mind. The subjective and the objective aspects of the chain of causation are then taken care of.

We must conquer our field of action. Objectively we must do our work perfectly, skilfully. Then it does not create any disturbance in the mind. The highest skill in action, combined with a subjective attitude of non-attachment, brings freedom.

I am reminded of an incident. I once went to see Mahatma

Gandhi. He was, as usual, busy spinning. He was also dictating to his secretary a very important article for *Young India,* of which he was editor. It was in answer to a challenge of Lord Birkenhead. He was also talking and joking with those who were sitting near him. And within ten minutes he was to catch a train to go on a lecture tour. All of his activities were perfect; he was calm, happy, and free. Mahatma Gandhi was a great karma yogin.

When you do your work to serve your higher Self, or to worship your God, or just for the sake of work, without any desire to reap its results for yourself, you will find that even the objective side of the work will manifest more perfection than otherwise. Moreover, in your heart you will remain filled with feelings of happiness, calm, and peace. You will be carried higher and higher in your consciousness by that wonderful uplifting current of unselfishness. The strongest chain that binds us to the pillar of ignorance is selfishness.

If you can work for the love of all, for the love of the Self which is present everywhere, and for the love of God, your work will be converted and consecrated into the most powerful form of spirit• ual exercise. You do not have to go to the Himalayas or practise any other yoga for the attainment of spiritual realization.

A karma yogin is a man of action, heroic and bold. He believes more in conquest than in avoidance. "Face the brute, don't flee from him," is the motto of his life. He is a born fighter and his fight is against the forces of attachment and selfishness. No matter whether he sweeps the streets or rules a kingdom, he seeks to do his work perfectly.

The secret of handling anything is to handle it with mastery. Be an expert.

You must know how to live in the world. If you want to play with snakes you must know how to charm them. Otherwise the snakes will bite you and end your life. Through karma yoga you learn the "charms" by which you can control the "snakes" of this world!

Karma yoga teaches the art of living.

All the yogas require that an aspirant follow certain disciplines. Sometimes these are rather difficult to observe. The requisites for following the path of karma yoga may be simply stated; but the implications are deep and far-reaching.

The three requisites for this path are: sincerity, steadiness, and discrimination. One must be *sincere* to the very backbone. Only a sincere person can develop the necessary persistence and tenacity that will keep him going. This is a great quality, to be sincere in the endeavour, without any ulterior motive, with no desire for results, with no attachment. *Steadiness* is a necessary quality of character. Only with it are you able to stick to the ideal through all the failures and the obstructions you will meet with. *Discrimination* is also essential for a student in any of the paths of yoga. Without it, the foundation cannot be laid.

An aspirant must become strong in these three. One should not become impatient and give up the endeavour just because of a setback now and then. If you are unsteady and always running after some new idea, something to pamper your ego, you will not get very far in any of the yogas.

A city school teacher once got tired of his job. He took a fancy to farming. He thought it would be wonderful to live close to nature, to hear the songs of the birds and to make his living directly from the bosom of Mother Nature. So he resigned his job in the city and bought a farm. But being ignorant of farming methods, he could not raise a crop the first year. The second year there was a flood which washed away the little he was able to raise. The third year there was a drought which burnt up all his plants. With all his savings gone the school teacher was very disillusioned. "Enough of this!" he said, and was back in the city looking for a job again. But a farmer who is one by profession cannot quit, whether there is flood or drought, and so he gains in the long run.

A student of yoga should be like the professional farmer and not allow anything—fire, flood, drought, or whatever—to interfere with his persistence in following the ideal. If he does not set his mind to anything else, he will succeed. But if he is just a fanciful amateur, he will not get far.

Very few can hold on to one ideal for the sake of the ideal itself. We follow a line of action, weaving into it, as we go along, a dozen different desires. If a single one fails, the whole fabric is ruined. A karma yogin works with the *single* motive of carrying himself and his work to the highest state of perfection. His constant meditation is: "I am going to stick to this one ideal, no matter what happens to me. Even if the whole world oppresses me, I shall not falter. If all praise me, I shall not be elated. So-called success or failure mean nothing to me. I want to work as an experiment to attain subjective perfection, and unless and until the goal is achieved I shall not stop. I shall not give up!"

In yoga, an aspirant is called an adhikari. An adhikari is a person with a specific capacity. Specific capacity or skill is inherent. It has been acquired in a previous incarnation. The adhikari in karma yoga is viewed from three aspects:

1) Willingness, simple willingness, not complex or subservient. This is called *arthitwa.*

2) Capacity or capability. In this, due consideration must be given to such conditions as health, background, resources, and so on. This is called *samarthya* is Sanskrit.

3) The absence of obstructing conditions, such as opposition from others, dependents who have to be looked after, and so on. This is *apratishedha.* It is very important to take care of this factor. Then the previous two will round out successfully.

Among karma yogins there are the "fast, medium, and slow" adhikaris. But a man must adhere to his ideal in his own way, without being influenced by what others are doing. A spirit of competition is a hindrance to progress in spiritual life. If you are a slow adhikari, you will not become a fast one by feeling jealous of someone else who seems to be ahead of you. The human mind is so competitive! One does not mind driving five miles an hour if someone else on the highway is not going fifty. But in spiritual life competition is most dangerous.

Human nature is composed of three basic qualities, or gunas, which we have already mentioned. Analyze yourself and find out which guna is most prominent in your nature. Each must work from wherever he finds himself at the present time. What someone else is doing is "none of your business." Each must adhere to his own path. He will reach the goal much quicker than if he is always bothering about what others are up to.

Humanity generally may be considered as falling into three types: (1) Those who are spiritually asleep and unaware of any purpose in life other than the satisfaction of the senses; (2) those who are beginning to wake up, to become aware of a higher, spiritual ideal and struggle to reach it; and (3) those who are fully awakened and who are living the ideal.

Sri Ramakrishna described these three types in this way:

The fishermen cast their nets into the water. They are filled with fish. Most of the caught fish are quite happy, being unaware of what will happen to them. They do not know that they are trapped. Others struggle to get out of the net, while still others leap out of it to freedom. We are like fish caught in the net of the world; in the net of karma, of cause and effect.

The majority of mankind, of course, will be found in the first group. If you think you belong to the second category you should make every effort to reach the goal in this very incarnation, in this very life. However, we should never have a word of condemnation for those who are still playing at the game they call life. Most are working out a heavy load of karma. Sri Ramakrishna told a humorous story about such persons.

Some fisherwomen went to the market and sold their fish. As they were walking home with the empty fish baskets on their heads, they were overtaken by a storm. Dark clouds covered the sky, and rain suddenly came down in torrents. The fisherwomen saw a house in the distance. They ran there for shelter and breathlessly entered the compound. They found themselves in a beautiful garden. When they knocked at the door of the house, the gardener's wife asked them to come in out of the storm. They hurried in, leaving their fish baskets outside the door.

The gardener's wife helped them to get dry and when the storm did not abate she gave them a room in which to pass the night. It was such as they had never seen before, for they were very poor. They lay down, but in the midst of this great comfort they found they could not sleep, even in such beautiful beds!

One of the fisherwomen said to her friend: "What's the matter with me? I can't sleep. The smell of these flowers is awful!"

Then with sudden inspiration she said, "I know what!" She jumped out of bed, ran outside and picked up the fish baskets. She sprinkled some water on them and brought them inside the bedroom. The aroma of fish filled the room and the fisherwomen fell happily asleep. The sound of their snoring soon filled the house!

When people have a great deal of karma to work out they are not ready to accept better things. They cling to those things that seem to give them happiness, the things they are used to.

People often complain and blame fate or God for the position they find themselves in. We may think that God is whimsical in granting favourable conditions to some and denying them to others. We think he is partial in granting his grace. It may seem that God is like a little child standing at the corner with a bag of candy in his hand. Someone asks him for a piece and he says, "No, I won't give you any!" To another he says, offerings a piece of candy, "Sir, do you want a piece of my candy?"

We do not know the karma of each individual, so we blame God for it all!

There was once a devout man who was practising spiritual disciplines. He had arranged a seat for meditation under a big tree in a forest. He sat down to meditate, but after a while he heard the roar of a tiger. Frightened, he got up and ran away. Meantime, a robber had been hiding in the woods watching the man sitting at his meditation. Seeing him run away he thought, "I wonder what would happen if I sit there and try to meditate? Let me try."

He sat down and closed his eyes as he had seen the other man do. Suddenly, a luminous Being appeared before him and asked: "What do you wish? I will give you any boon you want." The robber was astonished at this. He asked, "I have only one wish. Please tell me why I should be given any boon at all. I am not a devotee. Just out of curiosity I took this seat, after your devotee ran away in fear of the tiger."

"You think you are not devotee, but you do not know your past lives. I do. Your karma has now run its course," said the divine Being. "Now, I grant you spiritual illumination!"

None of us know how much good karma is behind us. It may bear fruit any day.

3

EACH individual has been born with a special bent of character that forms the main current of his life. We must discover how our minds flow in the current of life, and where our minds find their most natural enthusiasm. By taking into consideration our aptitudes, inclinations, and tendencies it is possible to find a field of action suitable to our particular nature where we may follow the path of least resistance in our work. This will minimize obstructions, thereby assisting us in unfolding our inner perfection. In Sanskrit this is called the theory of *swadharma*. *Swa* means "one's own," while *dharma*, from the root *dhri*, means "that which sustains"; that is, one's individual law that guides the developments of one's potentialities.

One's swadharma may be determined by taking into account several considerations. First, sex and heredity. One's swadharma is first established by one's being born a man or a woman. The duty of one is not the duty of the other; though nowadays the fields of their activities may overlap considerably. Each is great in his or her own sphere. There is no need for competition between the sexes. From your ancestors your have inherited certain tendencies. These are to be considered under the influence of heredity. Find out what the dominant field of your ancestors was. Find out what their main characteristics were.

You should also take into consideration the environment in which you were born and brought up. This includes your economic, social, religious, cultural and educational background.

In Hindu psychology we find emphasis on the importance of tendencies, aptitudes, and talents with which a person is born, more from the point of view of his past attainments, rather than from heredity, though heredity is also carefully considered. As we believe in reincarnation we also believe that a child is born with a certain karma carried over from previous lives. This karma, we believe, lies in a potential state in his sub-conscious mind, and influences, consciously or unconsciously, his present life. These tendencies which may not yet be expressed in the character may be discovered by psychological analysis. The karma a person has been born with is made up of the sum total of impressions he has received in previous lives and retained in the bottom layer of his consciousness. These are called *samskaras*. By analyzing the samskaras, one's potentialities may be ascertained. These may also be discovered by intuition. Intuition, however, is often found to be mixed with bias, although it really can be a great revealer.

Therefore, your swadharma, or that individual law governing the development of your individual potentialities, may be discovered by considering your sex, heredity and environment, and by psychological analysis and intuition. In selecting the field of your activity, it is essential to examine and study your swadharma. Find out what your swadharma is, in what line of activity you will be able to excel, in what field you will find the least resistance. Ask yourself, "In what field can I seek perfection most easily?" Choose carefully. And do not go into a field of action only for the sake of money, prestige, or fame. That will not lead you towards inner perfection. From the subjective point of view, it will spoil all your works.

Of course, you can work at any activity and still practise karma yoga. But in some you will find greater obstructions than in others because you lack certain capabilities. Find a field where the work fits your qualifications, where it suits your temperament, and where you can "fall in love" with it. Then your work will be just as good as worship.

Today, people have spread their energies over a wide range of activities. But you cannot do everything and do it all well, so it is better to specialize in a field in which you excel. Let one occupation create the dominant note in your life; then harmonize a variety of notes into a symphony. Modern life is inclined to be more extensive than intensive—a heterogeneous conglomeration of odd occupations. Emphasize one activity, through which you may reach perfection. Even if it is necessary for you to work in a field outside your swadharma, a spiritual attitude towards the work can be maintained; but it is more difficult. However, inner poise can be achieved in any field of endeavour.

The Bhagavad-Gita considers work from five different aspects, each of which must be perfected. I call it the "pentagon of success." First, the "field of action," the site. In Sanskrit this is called *adhishthana*. Second, there is "the doer," the agent, the *karta*. Third "the equipment," the instruments and implements necessary for the work. This is called *karanam* in Sanskrit. The fourth aspect is "the accuracy of the endeavour," the proper expenditure of effort or energy needed to do the work. In Sanskrit this is *cheshta*.

Before giving you the fifth side of the "pentagon," I should like to discuss these four items. Every activity is conducted in some field. If you go into a business enterprise without giving due consideration to the field, you may meet with awful failures. The field of action has to be determined from all possible angles in order to avoid obstructions and trouble late on. We should know what to expect.

In considering the doer of the work, the agent, we have to

understand his fitness, or lack of it, for the specific work. We
have to consider the capacity of the adhikari, the aspirant.
Herein comes the theory of swadharma again, the individual's
aptitude and ability as regards a particular work. There is another
very important point regarding the adhikari. In under-taking
any work the adhikari, first of all, must have faith in himself. In
Sanskrit, sraddha means more than faith. It means faith that
the inner perfection is within you and that you have the capacity
to unfold it. You have to believe that you are capable of surmount-
ing a whole mountain of difficulties, if necessary, to achieve your
goal. Believe that the divinity within you is going to express the
highest degree of beauty, utility, and perfection in your work. Do
not doubt it, even for a moment. Know that the strength is within
you. Assert that you have the power, that you have all the means.
Say to yourself, "I will get into action by means of my own endeavour." If today it appears that there is nothing you can depend
upon, if the whole world seems to be raised in opposition against
you, believe in that perfection which is within you. Try to cultivate
that faith in yourself. Do not be disgrunted because there is a little
obstruction or because a few waves of disappointment come your
way. Don't be a coward. Be bold. You have to have such
faith in yourself, and also in your field. This faith we call sraddha.

There must also be ways and means for the agent to act.
Sraddha alone is not quite enough. We have to consider the
discipline, education and training the adhikari has had for the
specific field of endeavour. A man must be trained in the line of
work he wants to pursue. He must learn his "business," whatever
it may be.

As far as other people are concerned, consider them also as
agents. All friends are not just friends; and acquaintances are
not just acquaintances.

Next are the implements or tools connected with the activity.
We have a slang saying in India: "He has no sword or shield,
yet he wants to be a soldier." So, if you want to be a soldier get
hold of your sword and shield and keep them clean, bright and
efficient. Take care of the instruments and then endeavour to use
them. For perfection in any field, the condition of the equipment must be given careful consideration.

Suppose a great singer is giving a concert and the piano is
out of tune. The whole performance will be ruined. The singer

will be completely frustrated and the audience thoroughly displeased. It may even demand its money back! All because the singer, the main doer of the action, did not see to the condition of the necessary instrument.

It may be interesting to know that in India the implements and tools of various trades are treated with reverence. It is not uncommon to see people show great respect for the instruments used in their particular field. In the annual ceremony known as *Vishwa-karma puja,* where God as the Designer, the Architect, of the universe is worshipped in an image, the tools are laid by the tradesmen before the image and His blessings upon them invoked.

The fourth aspect, accuracy of the endeavour, the proper expenditure of effort or energy in accomplishing the work, is considered from three angles: excess of expenditure, lack of expenditure, and misapplication of the expenditure of energy. Accurate effort means to "hit the nail on the head," using not too much energy or too little. Extravagance in the use of energy is unnecessary and points to defects in character, such as are associated with the quality of rajas which we discussed in connection with the three types of adhikaris. Shortage or lack of expenditure of energy or effort is due to mere laziness or dullness, or to misunderstanding of the nature of the work and its requirements. This is associated with the quality of tamas. The misapplication of the expenditure of energy is caused by lack of judgment or imbalance.

All of these have to be analyzed, adjusted, and corrected, so that we may do our work with the maximum of excellence and the minimum of energy. Work that expresses a maximum of beauty and utility with a minimum of effort is to be considered successful. When work is done with the attitude of manifesting the highest perfection through the particular work, it must be done skilfully. A karma yogin knows the skill of adapting his work and expressions according to the time, place, and environment. This is adaptability.

The fifth side of the "pentagon" of success is really the most important. Without it, even though the other sides have been taken care of, we cannot be sure of success in our endeavour. Our endeavour is not just to work to gain material success. We want to attain perfection through our work. Both the objective and the subjective sides of our work are important. This fifth item, therefore, is of paramount importance.

Some people call this fifth item destiny, fate or just luck. But, whatever it is, we have to take cognizance of it because it does have a bearing on our activity and we have no control over it. Emerson translated the Sanskrit word, *daiva,* into a beautiful expression—"the unscheduled ingredient." We always have to keep a wide margin for this unseen influence. Recognition of this fifth item makes for success in any endeavour. After having taken full care of the first four items, if there is still obstruction in our work, we have to surrender our will to that. For success in your work always keep a wide margin for the "unscheduled ingredient." Greater calmness, deliberation and steadiness are gained if allowance is made for this. Moreover, the acknowledgement of the existence of this unseen element curbs our vanity, selfishness. and attachment. These obstacles, and many more to our spiritual development will be eliminated if we recognize and make allowance in all our plans for this item of daiva, the fifth side of the "pentagon" of success.

We aspire so many things in life. But aspiration should be formed as the result of a good deal of consideration, and with a good deal of margin. If you know what you really want to be, you must experiment and then aspire after your ideal, taking into consideration all ramifications. Do not be carried away by your surroundings. The habits of our neighbours carry us away. Is it always what others have and do that *I* must have and do? Let us establish our aspirations only after careful consideration. What we really want to do is to go beyond aspirations. If there is always as aspiration in front of us, we cannot be happy. Determine just exactly what will bring fulfilment to your life. That requires disciplined thinking.

We talk about success in our life's work, and there are many people who want to attain that by some trick. They do not have the patience to go through the disciplines that are necessary. They are always looking for a short cut. But let me tell you, there is no short cut—absolutely none—to real success. Of course, you might attain what you think is phenomenal success in some line of activity; but eventually even that success will create failures in your spiritual life. Without the proper subjective attitude towards your work, no amount of objective success will have meaning. The disciplines of thought and action, which will manifest inner perfection in your work, must be gone through. *Self-consciousness has to be thoroughly renovated.*

There are three different stages through which an aspirant on the path of karma yoga advances. The first stage is that of self-purification. Your aim is to attain the highest spiritual perfection by means of your work. Therefore, you look upon all your work as a subjective process of cleansing, of purifying your self-consciousness. If you can maintain the right subjective attitude towards your work, you will never have any complaint against it, or the amount of work you have to do. The more work you do, the more will your consciousness be purified. You will not have any attachment to your work, either. Praise or blame will not concern you, because your work is being done *for your own benefit,* as a means of purifying your self-consciousness.

As you proceed, you will find your obstructions are gradually being minimized, and your work is beginning to manifest skill and efficiency. As self-consciousness becomes purer, divinity begins to shine out of all your activities, and perfection comes to your work. If you do work in the form of service, in this spirit of self-discipline or self-purification, layer after layer of more subtle obstructions will be shed. Your horizon will broaden. You will realize yourself present everywhere, in all different shapes and forms. Then the natural motive-force of your life will be to do good, for no reason at all, but because you cannot help it. Goodness becomes your nature. You begin to feel the presence of the Divinity in every being in the universe. Whatever you do becomes an act of worship.

When you have gone through these stages, you live in a state of constant bliss. There is no unhappiness possible for you—and no happiness. It is all supreme bliss, far above happiness and unhappiness. Selfishness has dropped away from you; and when that happens, ignorance disappears. You realize your higher Self, above all activity, the Witness of all, and you hold your consciousness in that Self. You know that in activity or in rest, in life or in death, your real Self has no concern. That is the samadhi of karma yoga.

The samadhi of karma yoga is qualified by the words, *sthita-prajna.* It is called sthita-prajna samadhi, which means "a process of steady wisdom." You may refer to Chapter II, verses 55-72, of the Bhagavad-Gita, for a discussion of the general characteristics of a man of sthita-prajna samadhi.

I may tell you that there are seven characteristics which distinguish a sthita-prajna from an ordinary worker. (1) He is free from desires. The only motive-force behind his work is to be able to realize his Witness Self in and through all his activities. (2) He is non-dependent. He does not depend upon any external forces, such as persons, time, or environment, as an ordinary worker does. His inspiration, his happiness, and his peace of mind come from *within himself.* (3) He is even-minded. He is neither elated by success nor depressed by failure in his activities. He keeps an even mind through all the "ups and downs" of his work. (4) He is free. He may go anywhere, do anything. But he is never attached to his actions. *He is free.* (5) He has complete control over his senses. He is the master of his senses, not their slave. (6) He is always cheerful and is a source of joy to all of those who come in contact with him. (7) He enjoys the realization of his higher Self throughout his life and activities. He realizes that he is not the doer; he is the Self, the Witness. A sthita-prajna keeps his consciousness on that higher Self. Therefore, he finds inaction in all action.

The ideal of the karma yogin, as we have discussed before, is to work so that his work does not bind him to the wheel of karma. When work is done in the spirit of service, that karma is no karma; it does not bind one. Karma yoga tinged with bhakti, or bhakti yoga permeated by the ideal of karma yoga, is suited to our modern needs. In fact, no matter what yoga you are following, as far as your actions are concerned, the ideal of karma yoga is essential. All must work. Let your work be service, worship. Then you will not become attached to it. All your activities will be an offering to your highest Ideal.

That is a very practical and simple application of karma yoga which anyone may follow in his life. The bhakta wants to realize the presence of his beloved God everywhere; the karmi strives to realize his oneness with the Self of all. Both want to realize God. The easiest way to do so is to look upon all your actions as service, or worship, to the God of your heart or the Self of all. Find Him in all. Serve Him, worship Him. Your little self will then wither away. Your actions will not be bound by selfishness and your activities will not bind you to the wheel of karma.

In the following lines of Swami Vivekananda's poem, "To a Friend," is contained the mantram of karma yoga:

These are His manifold forms before thee.
Rejecting them, where seekest thou for God?
Who loves all beings without distinction
He indeed, is worshipping best his God.

God is present in all people. Find Him in the poor and the hungry. Offer Him a piece of bread. There are sick and hungry people everywhere, even in your own home. Serve God in them. If you saturate yourself with the ideal of service, you will find Him everywhere.

Swami Vivekananda established a new epoch in service. He inaugurated a new spirit for the service of the Living God.

Regard yourself as an instrument for the service of God, maintaining this attitude towards the world of the non-self: "God is manifest in all beings, in all things." Let worship be synonymous with service.

4

WHAT we need is a philosophy of right action, right thinking, and right living. Spirituality is not attained by paying lip service to abstruse philosophical theories; it is not gained by dabbling in metaphysics or by nibbling at spiritual teachings. That results only in indigestion! Spirituality is achieved by living and putting into practice the great principles of religion. Therefore, I do not talk much on intellectual matters; and I *refuse* to preach so-called "big" philosophy. Philosophy has to be lived, not displayed or talked about. What does it matter if there is one god or twenty thousand gods in your life? What difference does it make if Brahman and the human soul are one or distinct? Perhaps this will shock you, but I am not here to entertain or to flatter. If your philosophy does not come down to help you in the struggles of your ordinary daily life, does not make the spiritual path clearer to you, it only pampers the ego. And the first step in spiritual life is to deflate that balloon of the ego! I ask you, are you better because of your study of philosophy? Do you conduct yourself in daily life with more harmony, more love, and more understanding? Are you becoming less full of self, less aggressive, more tolerant and loving to all? If so, your study of philosophy has become fruitful. But if it has raised another wall around you, distinguishing you from others whom you look down upon, I tell you, my friends, your study of philosophy has been futile—worse than futile!

So, I shall teach and preach until the last day of my life, not. so much of bombastic philosophy but the practical philosophy of *right living*, the philosophy that makes us better men and women, capable of reaching the highest goal of spiritual life. I shall preach the message of universal love, of the appreciation, understanding, and assimilation of a broad, universal principle that can be lived in our day-to-day life. That will be my song, the burden of my song. If you are wondering where such a practical philosophy can be found, I tell you with all sincerity that it is in India's philosophy of karma and reincarnation, of the divinity of the human soul, of the potential purity and equality of all beings, and of the freedom of choice of one's own spiritual path— the harmony of all religions. This is the philosophy that has to be lived. In earlier times, these grand principles were the guiding force of Indian life; but for many reasons India has largely forgotten them. Still, though they have been forgotten by many, and relegated to the realm of "big" talk by others, this is the philosophy that is sustaining India and will continue to sustain her. And it is the philosophy that can save the world from competition, strife, discontent, hatred, war—and total destruction.

A picture very often comes before my eyes in contemplation. I see the Ancient Mother of the universe seated on Her throne of glory surrounded by all the things that make life successful: love, power, beauty, efficiency, peace, and spiritual understanding. She holds in her hands a beautiful casket of gold, inlaid with many precious jewels. Within the casket is the most brilliant diamond imaginable, thousands of times more brilliant than the famous Kohinoor diamond. The Divine Mother has two sons, and She says to them: "My sons, I give you these as your heritage. Take care of them and all will go well with you."

After some time, for some reason or other, the two brothers fell into a disagreement. They decided to separate and divide their inheritance, the beautiful container and its precious diamond. One brother, fascinated by the beauty of the casket, claimed it for himself. The other brother said, "Brother, you can have the casket; *I* want the diamond." So one took the casket and the other the diamond.

The one who took the casket was able and efficient; he did

everything possible to please his artistic sense and that of his friends. The casket became the central part of his life and he surrounded it with ·everything that beauty, art, and efficiency could produce.

The brother who took the diamond hid it, so that no thieves could find it. Though he lived in poverty, he was satisfied with the knowledge that he had the most precious diamond in the whole world. Though there was not a single sign of beauty or prosperity about him, he had the consciousness that "I am the owner of a precious jewel that can purchase the whole world!" That consciousness kept him alive. He had nothing else to desire, so he had peace. He had That, attaining which one becomes immortal and goes beyond all suffering, though his bliss lacked beauty, constructive ability, efficiency, and phenomenal power.

I present the picture of these two brothers to you. One is active and energetic and has built everything of beauty and utility around the casket, the container, but he has not taken the trouble to see if the container could contain anything. What is a container without the contained? He accomplished many wonderful things, no doubt, inspired by that beautiful container. But is he really happy? Yes, it is good to have a beautiful container, a body. Adorn it as you like, beautify it as you will. But have you given consideration to whether the container could *contain* anything? Have you ever taken the trouble to see *what is within you*? A container is not to be worshipped for its own sake. Find that diamond! Unless that priceless diamond is found in the container, you will never be really happy; you will never find peace.

We could address these words to the other brother: "Do not merely talk about that priceless jewel you have hidden away. Remove it from its hiding place, let its brilliance shine out through all your life's work. Hold it in your hand, *feel* that you have it, and let the world know that you are the possessor of a great spiritual truth!"

My friends of the West, you have the container and you have embellished it and surrounded it with all that is efficient, practical, and satisfying to the senses. But know that it contains that precious diamond; know that within you is the spark of divinity. Find it, and reach the goal of life. And my brothers of the East, you may know that you have the precious jewel; but it can only shine in all its brilliance if it is taken out of its hiding place and installed once again in that beautiful container, given to you by the Divine Mother. These, then—the priceless jewel, the Divinity within, and the practical means to realize and express it—must not be separated. The reunion of these two brothers can bring into existence a new type of humanity and spiritualize the whole of life. That, my friends, would be the salvation of the human race.

V
A SUMMING UP
I.

LET us now review the aims of the four yogas. According to jnana yoga, phenomena are only an appearance; the self is nothing but Brahman, the only Reality. The method of this path is to remove maya, the veil of ignorance, by discrimination, and thereby be free and illumined. It is the "royal road of reason."

Raja yoga states that individual consciousness is nothing but Pure Consciousness. Due to agitations within the individual consciousness, it appears separate and limited. The method is discipline, concentration, and meditation to calm these agitations which distort consciousness and prevent perfection from manifesting itself.

Bhakti yoga holds that it is the apparent separation of the individual self, or soul, from its divine source that causes its present imperfection. Union with the divine source is attained by purifying the ego and directing our emotions solely to God.

Karma yoga states man's perfection is disturbed by his desires, by the setting in motion of the wheel of causation. Neutralization of karma is the method. When the thread of causality is burnt, perfection manifests itself.

Any one of these yogas prescribed for the different human psychological types, if followed to its logical conclusion, will lead to the highest spiritual realization. We rarely find, however, a person who is a *pure* type. The fact is that aspirants *lean* more towards one of the yogas than the others, due to certain natural, inborn tendencies, or samskaras. And today, life is so complex that specialization in just one of the yogas is neither practical nor possible. For instance, where is the man who can be a real jnani? Where is he who can honestly say: "I will sit here and *deny the existence of everything!*"? Today, it is necessary to combine the yogas. The teachings of the yogas should be harmoniously blended in order to develop in us a well-balanced spiritual character.

Swami Vivekananda said: "I want to preach a *man-making* religion." And he compared the yogas to a bird. "Three things," he said, "are necessary for a bird to fly—the two wings and the tail as a rudder for steering. Jnana [knowledge] is the one wing, bhakti [love] is the other, and [raja] yoga is the tail that keeps up the balance."

My criticism of the four yogas, if they stand alone, is this: intellect alone is *stony;* psychic phenomena alone are *spooky;* emotion alone is *sticky;* action alone is *shaky.* We must beware of these four "S's"! We must harmonize our intellect, intuition, emotion, and action.

Now, how are we to combine the yogas? Begin the day with raja yoga. Prayer and meditation will give you an undercurrent of poise like the lingering sound of a bell. Strike the "bell" again throughout the day as often as possible, even at work. Whenever you have time to yourself, be a raja yogi. The disciplines of raja yoga develop tenacity and strengthen the will; and they gradually bring consciousness to a state of tranquillity. Close the day, again with raja yoga, with concentration and meditation, eradicating all undesirable concepts that have clung to your consciousness during the day's activities.

Be a bhakta in your contact with others. See God in everything and offer worship to Him. You can worship God with flowers or with a broomstick. Establish Him in your home, in your life. Make Him your constant companion. Know that life is the expression of that Divinity. It is He who makes it lovable, makes it livable. With every breath feel that it is He. Nurture and cultivate bhakti in secret, in your heart. Weep for your God. Then dry your tears and "powder your nose" before you go out to face the world. Do not make a display of your devotion; that is cheap sentimentalism. Discipline in bhakti is very necessary.

In the field of action be a karma yogi. Work for the sake of work. Let your work be your worship. Always remain unattached to your work and do not let any desire creep in. "Throw self overboard" is the slogan of karma yoga. In person be like a "colourless colour," one that can take on any colour; be a perso· nality as fluid, as colourless, as water which can fit into any environment. Water takes upon itself the colour and dimensions of the vessels in which it is contained, but pour it out of the container and it is its natural self again, colourless and without shape.

The mind should be like that—ready to attach and ready to detach. If you set a red rose in front of a crystal, the crystal will appear to be red, like the rose. The colour of the rose is superimposed upon the colourless crystal. If you remove the flower, the red colour vanishes from the crystal. We must be like a crystal that can reflect any colour, any impression that is set before it, yet all the while know that the colour is not our Self. Be ready to reflect any "colour," any contact, but remain unattached to the contact.

In fact, the more we are able to reflect the colour of any contact the more successful that contact will be. The more harmony there will be between you and your environment. A personality that is always clashing with others is a personality "in the making." A crystal personality reflects every contact, but ever remains itself• It does not throw out any adverse vibrations. It is in complete harmony with all.

If you want to dye clothes in different colours in a bucket you have to wash the bucket thoroughly after each dyeing process. Otherwise your clothes will be spoiled. The dyeing process will not be successful. What does it mean? It means not to carry over one action or thought to another throughout the day. Renounce the "attachment" every time. Be ready to attach and equally ready to detach your mind from your actions. Wash the bucket clean every time!

A karma yogi knows the skill of adjusting his work and expressions according to the time, place, and the environment, always leaving room for the "unscheduled ingredient." Always consider your *attitude* in all your activities. Be perfect in both the subjective and the objective aspects of activity.

Last but not least, let your life be balanced and controlled by the intellect. Knowledge of fundamental principles gives you latitude and the power of adjustment. It synthesizes everything in life; it destroys any superiority complex. Jnana yoga develops discrimination and reasoning. The other yogas are held in form by it. It is the sustainer of the other yogas. Let your entire day, nay, your entire life, be controlled and guided by a disciplined and discriminative intellect, which to your life is like the rudder to a boat.

Sri Ramakrishna once said: "Tying up the knowledge of advaita [jnana] in the corner of your *dhoti* [wearing cloth] go out into the world and do as you please." That is, sustain all your activities with the knowledge of the fundamental principles of jnana. With that as the basis of your thinking you will not make any mistakes. Ramakrishna also said: "An expert dancer never takes a false step." By following the principles of the four yogas in your daily life, you will always be in touch with the divine force, at work or at play. You need never be very far from your Ideal

All the yogas aim at one thing: the attainment of perfection And we find that the root cause of all the obstacles to the attain ment of this perfection in yoga is the misconception we have of our ego-consciousness. From the viewpoint of jnana, the "I consciousness" has to be understood as an illusion, or a superim posed structure on the Self, and it must be eliminated through discrimination. When "I-consciousness" is eliminated, with it disappears the wordl. What remains is the Reality—Brahman.

In raja yoga the strongest and most basic agitation of con sciousness is the sense of "I-ness." When that has been subdued, divine Consciousness manifests itself.

In bhakti yoga the individual ego has to be purified and mini mized until it exists no more as such, but loses itself, melts into, as it were, the divine Consciousness conveived of as the Chosen Ideal.

In karma yoga, "I and mine" consciousness, which leads to desire and attachment, has to be relinquished. The "little I" as the doer of action has to be wiped out, and the "big I", the eternal Witness of all action, has to be realized as one's own Self. In all cases it is ego-consciousness with its various modifications that obstructs us from realizing our spiritual Ideal.

Let us consider this ego-consciousness. In connection with our study of jnana yoga, we had occasion to discuss the evolution of pristine Consciousness according to the analysis of the ancient sage, Kapila, and I mentioned that this had been accepted, for the most part, by the Vedanta philosophy. The differences between the two do not concern us at this point. We learned that Con sciousness (Brahman, in the language of Vedanta) projects all manifestation by the inscrutable power of maya. The evolution is in this manner: first, *mahat*, undifferentiated consciousness; then *buddhi*, universal intelligence; next *ahamkara*, individualized consciousness, the "I-am" consciousness in the individual; then *manas*, mind. From the mind follow the senses, the subtle sense objects, and the gross elements.

From this analysis we find that the "I-am" consciousness

begets the mind and all its faculties, as well as the external world of phenomena. Now, we may say that practices in yoga are intended to control consciousness at that point where it first becomes individualized, for it is the "I-am" consciousness that is the cause of man's obstacles to the realization of his real nature. We may note that according to this analysis the involution of this consciousness is in the reverse order. This will give you some idea as to the procedure of discrimination and meditation, of withdrawing the mind from the grosser to the finer modifications of consciousness. There are two directions the mind may take: effectward (outward) or sourceward (inward). By following the practices of yoga we go sourceward. Sri Ramakrishna once remarked: "We have to follow the same way out as we came in." This is very significant.

However, although yoga attempts to control and efface the individualized ego, this ego is very, very difficult to get rid of. It comes back, even after realization. So long as we are in a body we will have an ego-consciousness. Sri Ramakrishna often told his disciples: "Let the 'rascal' ego remain, but as the servant, the devotee of God."

We must cultivate the ego of devotion, the witness ego, or the ego of knowledge. Establish a definite relationship of your "I-am" consciousness with your Ideal. If you are a monist, you must strive to know that your "I" is not what it appears to be. It is Brahman, the Whole, and you must try to maintain this identity. If you are a dualist, establish a particular relationship with God, your highest ideal of perfection. After the words, "I am," utter a phrase that will connect you with that ideal. Say, "I am the child, the servant, the friend, the lover of my God." Establish a relationship and keep it foremost in your thoughts. If you try to stand alone in your "I am" consciousness you are in constant danger. If everything in this world fails you (and sooner or later it will) this one relationship with your God will never let you down. Depend on God. Then your life will be freed from attachment, freed from fear and from all the other things that make you feel small, miserable and insecure.

I might say that very few people can do without a personal conception of their Ideal. There was once a highly metaphysical sect in Japan. There were no ceremonies or temples. They believed that their egoes were like mirrors and that all they had to do was to keep the mirrors of their minds clean in order to reflect God. But, eventually, temples arose with large mirrors installed in them. Brushes were kept beside the mirrors and people would go to the temples and brush the mirrors, to symbolize the cleansing of their egoes! It seems that people cannot go on for long without ceremonies of some kind. However, it is wise to allow ceremonies to grow—with a little rationalization. This one was, at least, artistic!

Do not form a pet theory that divinity may be manifest in one way only. Light may be diffused in various ways. And do not slacken the search for truth. See the soul of goodness even in the vicious. Say to yourself, "I shall make no compromise of the truth, no matter in what form God appears." God sometimes wears a thick mask, but don't let that fool you. Keep a constant current of understanding flowing within you. Fall in love with God, but not with the masks He is wearing! Find God behind all the masks and be concerned with Him alone. Find freedom.

God may be conceived of in many ways. He may be personal or impersonal. Practise using the word, "relative," in ordinary conversation and you will find a broadmindedness unfolding within you. Do no think that the Absolute Principle is the only conception of God. Recognize the Personal Divinity as well as the Impersonal.

In the life of Sri Ramakrishna we find synthesis of all aspects of the Godhead, of all religious outlooks. He taught that different religions, different approaches to the Reality, are all relative. They are just different readings of the one Truth. None can be called better or poorer readings, but just *different* readings. The final Truth cannot be known or discussed. It can only be experienced. It remains absolute.

Ramakrishna once gave this illustration: "God is at the centre of a circle and we are all standing at different points on its circumference, looking at Him through hollow tubes. Each thinks that He, at the centre, is his goal. The Christian, Hindu, Mohammedan, and so on; the dualist, the qualified nondualist, and the monist—they all think that He, the ultimate Reality, is at the centre. But they are viewing Him from their respective positions on the circumference and they are seeing Him through their own, individual tubes. Now, if they all proceed by looking at their God in their own way, they are bound to meet at the same place —the centre of the circle. So, it is said: "The Goal is one; the paths many."

The secret is to proceed towards the centre by some path, any path, and not merely to stand still and dispute and argue, and find fault with everything and everyone except ourselves!

Scattered information on the subject of the yogas may be found even in the literatue of the Vedic age. The Sanskrit language expresses an ocean of learning. But there was no such thing as chronology in ancient India; that is accurate, 'scientific' chronology. At best, it is "shaky". This is due in part, perhaps, to the tendency of the Indian mind to emphasize principles rather than personalities. Therefore, it is sometimes difficult to ascertain the exact dates of people and happenings in ancient times. Although jnana yoga was expounded in ancient texts and brought to a supreme climax in the Upanishadic literature, it came to be associated with the great philosopher and saint, Sankaracharya, who lived in the eighth century. He firmly re-established the Vedanta philosophy after a thousand years of Buddhist influence. His interpretation of Vedanta remains today as one of the fairest flowers of philosophy the world has ever known.

Raja yoga, also of ancient origin, immediately brings to mind the great sage, Patanjali, who contributed the famous *Yoga Aphorisms*.

Great authorities on bhakti yoga were Narada and Sandilya, both of whom left works, entitled the *Bhakti Sutras*. Madhwa and Ramanujacharya were prominent exponents of the path of bhakti belonging to a later period.

Although no specific book is considered by scholars to be directly connected with Karma yoga this yoga is so important that it forms the theme of every yoga. (Some claim that the Bhagavad-Gita is a book on karma yoga.) The *Yoga-Vasishtha,* which contains 80,000 verses, is considered to be a great literary monument to karma yoga.

All the yogas have been dealt with in a masterly manner by Swami Vivekananda. If you are interested in going more deeply into the study of the yogas there is ample opportunity. But take the study in real earnest, with the intention of putting these grand principles into practice. Otherwise, you will only add to the already heavy load of knowledge you already carry on your shoulders.

A blessed ignorance is the end of all quests after knowledge, and this is where philosophy and religion begin. But even philosophy can only *convince* you of the truth. There must follow some practices to *unfold* the inner reality. Live it and feel it at every step of your life. Discover the path that suits you best and follow it, without losing time trying to impose your ideas upon others. Turn your mind "sourceward." Meditate on the consummation of life. Otherwise, life is just a futile process. Examine the so-called offerings of life that people run after so madly. Gradually, you will question the value of the conventional things of life. Begging at the door of sense objects, you will never fill your begging bowl. What is a penny worth if you have a million? What is the loss of penny, when you have a million? Let pennies come and go. Know the wealth of the inner Self.

2

THE practices and disciplines of the yogas are intended to bring the mind of the aspirant to a state of poise and steadiness. Under their influence, the obstacles to the unfoldment of inner perfection will be minimized. Without having attained that state of mental steadiness and calm, the student will find it difficult to follow any of the practices of yoga, much less to concentrate his mind or to meditate. An unsteady and uncontrolled mind is a liability, never an asset. It is of the utmost importance for the spiritual aspirant to attain a refined and calm state of mind.

We have previously discussed the gunas. All manifestation, including the consciousness of man, is characterized by these there modes of expression of prakriti. Sattva means a state of poise and tranquillity; rajas, activity, imbalance; and tamas, lethargy, inertia. Though all three of these gunas are present in man, one predominates over the others. We may consider a man's character and state of spiritual development from the point of view of the gunas under four headings: general characteristics and manners, outlook on religion and ethics; choice of food; habit of dress.

General characteristics and manners: A man dominated by tamas will be slovenly, inaccurate, careless, and clumsy. One, who is influenced by rajas will be over-enthusiastic, boisterous, changeable, unsteady and domineering. He in whom the state of sattva predominates will be calm, sure, compromising, steady, and true.

Outlook on religion and ethics: The tamasic man will be narrow and superstitious, full of fear, often cruel, and subject to compulsion and force. The rajasic man will tend to be bigoted, aggressive, self-righteous, superficial, and ostentatious. The sattvic man will have a broad, universal, and tolerant understanding. He will be all-loving, and accommodating to the beliefs of others.

Choice of food: The tamasic man will choose an immoderate diet. He will not particularly care if it is fresh or clean or health-giving. The rajasic man will like food that is over-rich, heavy and generally exciting and alluring to his senses. The sattvic man will choose wholesome, mild, fresh food in moderate amounts.

Habit of dress: The tamasic man will dress in a careless and slovenly manner, being disproportionate and even uncouth in his habit of dress, without aesthetic sense. The rajasic man will choose gaudy, colourful, exciting and immodest clothing. The sattvic man will dress in a clean, neat, unshowy and modest manner.

The procedure for the attainment of the perfection we strive for in the practice of yoga is to overpower a lower guna by a higher one, and eventually go beyond all the gunas. We know that the mind and body are interrelated. One influences the other. When the body is ill, the mind is disturbed. When the mind is depressed and dull, the body, too, reacts. Whether we like it or not, our outer habits have a great deal to do with our inner life. Even such a simple thing as dress can affect the mind.

Sri Ramakrishna gave two amusing illustrations of how outer actions and habits play upon the mind, and how they can change our character. He said that when a man dresses himself in fine clothes, like a dandy, he begins to sing the popular love songs of the day (Nidhu Babu's love songs). And he even thinks of carrying a fashionable walking stick and of playing cards! The Master also said that even if a weak and sickly man puts on high boots, he begins to whistle like an Englishman; and like him, even dashes up the stairs in great haste!

There are many stories in Hindu literature illustrating the effect which manners and dress have on the gunas. These are psychological facts. By making changes in our bodily habits, we are able to alter the moods of the mind. If we try to control the outer expressions of the gunas in our nature, the work of elevating the mind will be made much easier. The spiritual aspirant is to analyze himself and his habits very carefully and sincerely, and always strive through all his thoughts and actions to *appreciate*, to *feel,* and to *express* the highest principles of spiritual life. Discipline in all phases of life is absolutely essential.

The meaning of the three gunas for man, in so far as they have a bearing on his spiritual ascent, is that he has to rise to a state which is governed predominantly by the sattva principle. Then at last he must rise above all three of the gunas and become *tri-guna-atita* (the description of the state of perfection which is beyond the gunas). Let us take an illustration from the physical world. Water, in its usual state, is earthbound. It cannot ascend from its earthly boundaries until it is rarefied into steam. But once it becomes steam it easily rises in the sky where it is transformed into clouds, and then descends in the form of rain to fructify and bless the earth. We are like water. We have to strive to rarefy ourselves so that the ego in us vanishes and we merge in the Infinite, to the eternal good of all.

There are three great urges that bind man down to the lower forms of being. They are equally powerful and are always feeding one another. They are the sex urge, the taste urge, and the love of money. These have to be controlled by discipline.

Each mind is connected with every other mind and each mind is, therefore, in actual communication with the whole world. This has advantages as well as disadvantages, depending upon the state of spiritual unfoldment you have reached. If your mind is attuned to uplifting thought-forces, you draw in influences that will assist your spiritual growth. But, you have to build up your resistance against destructive thought-forces also. Train your mind to be antagonistic to undesirable concepts. Remember, habits are nothing but crystallized concepts and by exerting yourself you can alter your habits and develop a character which will express spiritual truths. One overcomes difficulties in spiritual life by determination, not by confusion. *Know* what you want to get, and it is yours. You have all the tools.

We think so much but do so little. Analyze yourself and find out why it is so. There are various things that interfere with the "doing" Perhaps you do not feel strongly enough about it. Or, if you do feel, perhaps you waste your emotion. Or perhaps you are engulfed by doubt. Some people are so constituted that they cannot reach conclusions. But the mind can be cultivated to reach conclusions quickly, and be right. If you really desire to accomplish anything, it is yours "for the taking." Everyone has the same amount of will. Develop it and use it.

Right conduct is one of the items in the Eight-fold Path propounded by Buddha. Conduct is such a vague expression, and yet such a deep one. It pervades every one of man's expressions. One can hurt another without talking, just by one's silent conduct. We all know this. One can do wrong without moving the body. Attitude determines conduct. A child, for instance, makes mistakes but does not offend us.

A man's conduct is the outcome of his attitude towards his inner being. What is your attitude toward yourself, toward other individuals, toward groups of people? Let your conduct, which should be guided by the right attitude, be worthy of your inheritance, worthy of the inner Divinity. Try to maintain the right attitude under all circumstances. Naturally, you will make many errors. Never mind. Errors are lights pointing to Him. Work, play, laugh—and pray that the veil will be lifted; your actions and conduct will be adjusted accordingly.

In spiritual pursuits we must have the boldness and courage to walk over the "royal road", the road of being and becoming, of hard struggle and labour. We know many things which, if rightly practised, would make our lives divine. But we lack the patience and perseverance to practise them. We have to fight our own battles as much as we have to eat our own bread. No one can do you any good by eating bread for you. If we know only one principle, and can carry that into practice, it will be enough to make our lives holy. The clearest and most open thing in the world is the means to attain divine life; but because of our passions and weaknesses we have covered that up with all sorts of "secret knowledge," and lots of other nonsense. The "open sesame" to spiritual life is the secret of being and becoming, of having the strength and courage to carry a thing into actual practice, no matter how simple and devoid of high-sounding and befooling name it may be. This is the "open secret," knowing which we can wake up from this long painful world-dream. There is no short-cut to that.

Truth is always simple. It is only falsehood that is intricate and complicated. Spirituality is simplicity. I find that many people are interested in yoga, particularly raja yoga. But most of them have a very odd conception of what it really is. Many think that it is something magical, like Aladdin's lamp, something that can bring them, without the least trouble, all the things they wish to enjoy. They learn a couple of postures and a few peculiar ways of breathing and right away they become Aladdins of the twentieth century, even without a lamp! To others it appeals as the builder of perfect health and enduring beauty. Do whatever you like, live any way you please, only learn some yogic tricks and then you are free from indigestion, headache, and overweight! And lo! Look into your mirror and see what magic charm your features radiate.

These are all complexes. Only when everything about a person has become simple can the Truth reveal itself in its simplest and healthiest form. It is weakness of the brain that gathers mystery around yoga. Yoga is not for the weak. What we want is mysticism without the "mist". I consider it my business to bring all types of "magic" into the penetrating light of knowledge, so that whatever is fake in them will vanish, and whatever is real and true will gain the precision of scientific knowledge. I therefore earnestly request you to cast from your minds all notions of mystery and magic regarding yoga. Spiritual unfoldment does not mean the achievement of any supernatural or magical powers. Far from it!

To keep your body strong, you direct four kinds of attention to it. You give it food; you keep it in good health; you exercise it; and you give it enough rest. Now, should not the mind demand the same attention from you? Poor mind, nobody pays any attention to it! It is time that man devotes equal attention to his mind. The mind needs nourishment. It needs to be kept clean. It must be properly exercised, and it demands sufficient rest. The practices of yoga furnish the mind with all of these. Without them, the mind grows weak and susceptible to many degenerating influences.

A healthy, concentrated, and disciplined mind focussed on any study, work, or endeavour, will give you more efficient results than an undiscipline, uncared-for mind can ever do. Achievements depend on practice in mental discipline.

In all branches of knowledge, the teacher stimulates past achievements in you. The gaining of knowledge is an unfoldment from within. The ego-consciousness of each person invests the subject with a special "colour." The individual (whether a spiritual aspirant or a student of worldly knowledge or science) must struggle until the ego has been cleansed, so that the light of understanding may *shine out from within*. This has been recognized by all teachers of yoga, and it may be applied to any field of study.

There are four "Golden Rules" for study in any field: (1) Use discrimination in selecting the material you are to study. (2) Read, study, and contemplate everything from cover to cover. (3) Do not let a single word, figure of speech, or idea pass until you are convinced that you know the author's meaning. Always try to get his viewpoint. (4) Reserve your right of free, consistent, logical judgement. Data are supplied by the author, but judgement must be strictly your own.

The reason why we do not get more results from our spiritual, or even from our intellectual, acquisitions is that we talk out more than we receive. We have to accumulate knowledge or spirituality before we can expend it. Silence should be cultured. Do not be in a hurry to show off your knowledge! Many spiritual aspirants get a few ideas and immediately want to teach others. That is merely the ego asserting itself. Gradually, as the inner Divinity unfolds and manifests itself, you may be able to help others by your talk. But until then, keep silent. Accumulate first. Then spirituality will radiate from you without your having to make an effort to express it. And another thing, always remember that it is God's power that is being expressed through you. Never think that you alone can do anything.

Give up vain and unnecessary argumentation. Half the literature of philosophy has suffered refutation by others. Don't get yourself involved in such a futile pastime.

Rituals, dogmas, statistics, and logic-splitting philosophy are all primary stages in religion. Real religion begins with *being and becoming.*

Two men once went into a mango grove. One started to enumerate the various types and species of trees and their fruit, and quoted eminent botanists to uphold his opinions. The other man quietly found the owner of the garden, who explained all about the mango trees and invited him to eat as many mangoes as he liked. When the men left the garden one man had a pile of statistics, but did not know what a mango really was. He did not have the time to taste a fruit. Only the man who ate the mangoes knew what mangoes were. Let us not spend our valuable time counting leaves and twigs and quoting authorities. Let us seek the Owner of the garden and eat mangoes!

What all the yogas teach is this: know God, realize Brahman. Know that whatever is done through the machinery of your body and mind is because of the omnipotence of God. No matter what your conception of God may be, it is that God, that Infinite Power, which is expressing itself through your "container". Do not pay much attention to the containers. Realize the *Substance* within, and you are free *now*.

We have heard enough talk. We have studied enough writings. Now let us be up and doing, for the *doing* is something that must be done!

GLOSSARY

abhisara—defiance of custom and environment for the sake of the beloved Ideal.

adhikari—a student who is competent to understand the highest spiritual truth after undergoing the essential spiritual disciplines.

adhisthana—the field of action.

advaitavada—nondualism. The school of Vedanta, the essence of philosophy and religion of the Vedas;the"perennial philosophy." Also simply *advaita*.

advaita Vedanta—see ADVAITAVADA.

agama—scriptural authority.

ahamkara—consciousness associated with ego or sense of "I".

ajatavada—strict monism or ADVAITA. The view that there is no manifestation, that all is a mere illusion.

anandamaya kosa—see KOSAS.

anishta parihara—action done in fear of achieving undesirable ends.

annamaya kosa—see KOSAS.

apratishedha—the absence of obstructing conditions, opposition from others, and so forth.

arthitwa—willingness to follow spiritual disciplines.

asana—one of the eight limbs of RAJA YOGA. Also a steady and easy posture mastered by the yogi to assist him in concentrating the mind.

ashta siddhi—the eight great yogic powers.

ashrama—a retreat for seekers of truth.

ashtanga yoga—RAJA YOGA, so called because it has eight parts or "limbs." These are: YAMA, NIYAMA, ASANA, PRANAYAMA, PRATYAHARA, DHARANA, DHYANA, and SAMADHI.

Atman—Pure Consciousness conceived as the individualized Self. ATMAN and BRAHMAN are one.

Atmasamarpanam—self-surrender to God; self-abnegation.

avidya—the veil of ignorance, both cosmic and individual, obscuring the true knowledge of the Self.

Y—14

bala samadhi—behaving like a five-year-old child while absorbed in God.

bhakti yoga—the path of devotion, through which ultimate Unity is experienced between the devotee and God.

bhava—an attitude of devotion towards the Ideal. There are, in all, six such attitudes of devotion: SANTA BHAVA, DASYA BHAVA TATA BHAVA, SAKHYA BHAVA, VATSALYA BHAVA, and MADHURA BHAVA.

bhava samadhi—the state of merging the individual consciousness into the ISHTAM with the help of a particular attitude.

brahmacharya—the necessary spiritual consciousness possessed by a student; the first stage of life in orthodox Hindu society. It also means purity of body and mind.

Brahman—the ultimate Reality, the Unity of all that exists. Indicated as Existence absolute, Knowledge absolute, and Bliss absolute.

buddhi—that form of consciousness or aspect of mind which discriminates between "this" and "not this".

chakras—centres of consciousness along the central spinal canal (sushumna). They are: *muladhara, svadhishthana, manipura, anahata, visuddha, ajna,* and *sahasrara.*

cheshta—activity or endeavour.

chinmaya—a subtle plane of consciousness.

chitta-vritti—ripples or waves occurring in the mind-stuff. A disturbed condition of mind.

dama—restraint of the external sense organs.

darsana sastra—philosophy and religion which teaches one to *see* things as they really are.

dasya bhava—the attitude of a servant to his master in BHAKTI YOGA.

dharana—retention of the concentrated power of the mind on the object of meditation. The seventh limb of YOGA.

dhyana—meditation; the constant flow of the power of the mind towards the object of meditation. The sixth limb of RAJA YOGA.

dinata—humility.

dvaitavada—the religion and philosophy of dualism.

garhasthya—the second stage of life in Hindu society; family life at home.

Gaudapada—a great seer of ancient India who forcefully advocated the AJATAVADA theory of ADVAITA VEDANTA.

Gita—the Bhagavad-Gita, one of the three great scriptures of the Hindus, the other two being the Brahma Sutras and the Upanishads.

Govindapada—disciple of GAUDAPADA and Guru of SANKARACHARYA.

granthi—literally a "knot"; the bondage of ignorance.

guna—one of three forms of energy or ways in which PRAKRITI is expressed. They are SATTVA, RAJAS, and TAMAS.

guru—in the highest sense of the term, an illumined spiritual teacher. It can also refer to anyone who teaches or professes to teach spiritual truths.

hatha yoga—a system of physical discipline that maintains the body in a clean and healthy condition.

Ishta Nishtha—unqualified devotion to the Ideal.

Ishta prapta—action done to avoid undesirable issues.

Ishtam—the spiritual Ideal of the aspirant.

Iswara—the ultimate Reality, viewed as Creator, Preserver, and Destroyer.

Iswarakoti—a person spiritually illumined from birth; companion of an Incarnation.

jagat—the universe of phenomena; the world of change.

japam—the repetition of a MANTRAM.

jiva—the individual self; philosophically speaking, Jiva is ATMAN identified with the KOSAS or sheaths of ignorance.

jivakoti—an ordinary being possessed of physical consciousness.

jnana yoga—the path of Knowledge, in which ultimate unity of subject and object is realized.

kalaha—quarrelling between lover and Beloved in BHAKTI YOGA.

Kapila—a very ancient sage; founder of the Sankhya system of philosophy.

Karana sarira—the causal body.

karma—actions, both physical and mental, and the effect of such actions.

karma yoga—the path or science of action in which every physical and mental act created by our personality finds its way to the universal Being.

karta—one who acts.

kosas (*pancha kosa*)—the five sheaths or covers, as it were, of the Self. The five are *annamaya kosa,* the outermost sheath or gross body; *pranamaya kosa,* the covering composed of the five vital forces; *manomaya kosa,* the covering of the mind; *vijnanamaya kosa,* the sheath of the intellect; and *anandamaya kosa,* the sheath of Bliss.

Kriyamana karma—the effect of actions being performed now.

Kundalini Sakti—the subtle spiritual power that ordinarily lies dormant at the base of the spinal column.

Linga sarira—Composed or seventeen component parts: five organs of perception, five organs of action, five vital forces, mind, and intellect: also called *sukshma sarira.*

madhura bhava—the attitude of a lover toward his Beloved in BHAKTI YOGA.

mahasamadhi—final liberation. It also may mean the giving up of the body while in the highest meditation.

mahat—undifferentiated, cosmic intelligence.

mana—pique or assumed indifference in BHAKTI YOGA.

manana—using the discriminative faculty of the mind to consider spiritual propositions given to the student.

manas—that form of consciousness which receives sense impressions and experiences sense objects.

manomaya kosa—see KOSAS.

mantram—a holy name or phrase given by a guru to a disciple, and intended for repetition in order to concentrate the mind.

maya—cosmic power, which veils the Reality and projects in its place something which is not the Reality. The world as seen in ignorance.

mayavada—the view that the Reality is covered by and projected as something other than it actually is.

medha—spiritual intelligence. The spiritual faculty which instills in an aspirant the desire to realize the Truth.

milana—union with the Ideal; nearness to the ISHTAM.

mithya—that which is unreal.

mumukshutwam—intense yearning for freedom from worldly bondage.

nidhidhyasana—constant meditation on the propositions taught and communicated to the student by SRAVANA AND MANANA. Constant contemplation of the goal.

nirvikalpa samadhi—the highest state of spiritual realization in which all limiting adjuncts have been removed and only awareness of the One, BRAHMAN, remains.

nishtha—tenacity in following spiritual practices.

niyama—the second limb of RAJA YOGA comprising the five observances.

Om—the mystic sound symbol of BRAHMAN, the Absolute (pronounced a-u-m).

paramahamsa—one who has attained to the highest realization of God.

paramarthika—absolute truth.

pisacha samadhi—behaving like a madman while absorbed in God.

prakriti—one of the two ultimate principles of the SANKHYA philosophy. Prakriti denotes the material principle of the universe which evolves as mind and matter.

pramana—that by which truth is established.

prameya—that which we want to prove.

pranamaya kosa—see KOSAS.

pranas—modifications of *prana*, the vital principle which sustains all life, which are concerned with the vital functions of the body. These are *samana*, assimilating energy, located in the stomach area; *apana*, expelling energy, located in the organ of excretion; *udana*, the uplifting energy; and *vyanas* the vital force which moves in all directions and pervades the entire body.

pranayama—fourth step in the discipline of RAJA YOGA which restores harmony and rhythm of breathing.

prarabdha karma—the result of karma initiated in past lives that must run it course; unalterable conditions.

pratyahara—centralization of the power of the mind; the fifth step in the eightfold path of RAJA YOGA.

pratyaksha—direct perception.

prema bhakti—unselfish love for the Ideal; the negation of self-interest in that love.

puja—ritualistic worship.

Purusha—one of the two ultimate principles of the SANKHYA philosophy. Purusha denotes the Self of or Pure Consciousness in every being.

purva raga—primary attachment in BHAKTI YOGA.

raganuga bhakti—worship with attachment to the Ideal.

rajas—that GUNA or form of energy·that expresses itself as restlessness and overactivity, leading to desire and attachment.

raja yoga—the path by which Unity is experienced within through the control of both internal and external forces.

Sat-chid-ananda—Existence—Knowledge—Bliss Absolute. The only known positive description of the ultimate Reality.

sakhya bhava—the attitude of a friend towards a friend in BHAKTI YOGA.

samadhana—steady concentration of the restrained mind on those forms of consciousness conducive to spiritual experience.

samadhi—the final point in YOGA when the PURUSHA realizes that it is separate from PRAKRITI; absorption.

samarthya—capability, as it is reflected in one's environment; state of mental and physical health etc.

samskara—the sum total of past impressions, caused by thoughts and actions, that remain in a subtle form in the subconscious and which may come to the surface in the present life.

sanchita karma—accumulated karma that is ready to take effect.

sandhya—that period when day passes into night and the night into day. These periods are considered particularly favourable for spiritual practices.

sankhya—one of the six systems of Hindu philosophy. Founded by KAPILA.

sannyasin—a Hindu monk. One who has renounced worldly life in order to realize the Supreme Reality.

sarsthi—a grade of Mukti or liberation with equal power or rank as the ISHTAM.

sarupya—a grade of Mukti with the same or similar form as the ISHTAM.

sattva—that GUNA which is the principle of tranquillity and peace.

A state of equilibrium achieved when free from RAJAS and
TAMAS.

satyam—Truth; Reality.

sayujya—constantly attached to the ISHTAM.

seva—service; especially service to God as worship of Him.

sama—restraint of the outgoing propensities of the mind.

Sankaracharya—8th century sage and seer of great renown, who
firmly reestablished the ADVAITA philosophy in India after a
thousand years of Buddhist influence.

santa bhava—the attitude of transcendent awe and reverence in
BHAKTI YOGA.

sarira—objectified covering of the ATMAN.

sushumna—according to RAJA YOGA, the hollow canal which runs
through the centre of the spinal cord.

siddhanta vakyam—concise, condensed, and final statement about
the ultimate Truth.

sishya—a student gifted with the essential spiritual qualities.

smaranam—constant remembrance of the Ideal.

salokya—belonging to the same sphere or region as the ISHTAM.

sraddha—a reasoned, firm faith in the instructions of the spiritually
illumined teacher.

sravana—hearing or listening to subjects that deal with the highest
spiritual goal.

srishti—projection or gradual unfoldment of the universe from
seed state; projection.

sthita-prajna—one of steady spiritual understanding; a man of
the highest wisdom.

sthula sarira—the gross body; most external covering of the ATMAN.

sukshma sarira—the subtle body, which, after death of the physical
body, forms the basis of a new physical body for an unillumined
soul. *See also* LINGA SARIRA.

swadharma—one's own individual law of development.

tamas—that GUNA or form of energy that expresses itself as inertia,
delusion. Lit. "darkness."

tanmatras—in SANKHYA cosmology, the subtle principles of the
five basic elements before their expression as ether, air, fire,
water, and earth.

tata bhava—the attitude of a child towards its parents in BHAKTI
YOGA.

tirthas—places of pilgrimage. Etymologically, the word means "that which enables one to swim over."

titiksha—not affected by the pairs of opposites such as joy and sorrow, pain and pleasure, etc.

tushti—self-satisfaction; an obstruction to progress in spiritual life.

unmatta samadhi—to act like a crazy or drunken man while absorbed in God.

upadhi—a limiting condition of the true Self.

uparati—cessation of external sense organs; a state where the mind does not react to stimuli.

upasana—to remain near the object of worship.

vaidhi bhakti—formal worship of the Ideal.

vaikuntha—a region without imperfection or defect; heaven.

vairagya—dispassion; renunciation.

vanaprastha—third stage of life in Hindu society, primarily characterized by contemplation and intensive spiritual study.

vatsalya bhava—the attitude of a parent to its child in BHAKTI YOGA.

vidya—true knowledge of the Self.

vijnanamaya kosa—see KOSAS.

vikaravada—the view that the Supreme Being has actually been transformed into the universe.

viraha—the acute sense of separation from the Ideal.

vishwa premi—one who loves the whole universe as God.

visishthadvaita—the religion and philosophy of qualified nondualism, which teaches that all creatures and nonliving matter are part of BRAHMAN.

vivartavada—the view that there is an appearance, but that the appearance is not the actual and final truth.

viveka—that intellectual power which discriminates between the real and the unreal.

vyavaharika—relative truth.

yama—the first of the eight steps of RAJA YOGA comprising the five practices.

yoga—1. A state in which the individual consciousness is merged with cosmic consciousness—as a water drop merges into a lake. 2. The method or methods to realize this state. 3. When capitalized, the path of RAJA YOGA.

INDEX

abhisara (defiance of custom), in
   bhakti yoga, 141
Absolute, the, 74
abstinence, need for, 101
Adbhutananda, Swami, quoted,80
action
   standard for good and bad, 159
   types of, 158-159
adhikari (aspirant), 129, 130, 172
   defined, 36
   qualifications of, 37
ahamkara, 23
ahimsa (non-injury), in *raja
   yoga*, 96
annamaya kosa (physical
   sheath), 23
aparigraha (non-acceptance of
   gifts), in *raja yoga*, 99-100
asana (posture), 95
   in *raja yoga*, 104-105
ashtanga yoga (*eight limbs*) in
   raja yoga, 95
aspirant (*adhikari*)
   bhakti yoga and, 129, 130
   karma yoga and, 172
Atman, 18, 23, 24
atmasamarpanam (self-surrender)
   136, 144
attachment, in *bhakti yoga*, 139
attitude in life, 188
austerity (*tapah*), in *raja yoga*, 101

Bhagavad-Gita, and work, 176
Bhagavata, 137-38
bhakta (lover of God)
   attitudes and goal of, 153-54
   relationship with God in
      after-life, 154-55
   view of death and, 154

bhakti
   abuse of powers of, 145-147
   as natural way, 147
bhakti worship, in Hinduism, 136
bhakti yoga
   defined, 126
   goal of, 126
   karma yoga and, 181
   summarized 186
bhava (attitude toward God),
   stages of, 131
bhava samadhi, 151, 152
bhavas, types described, 130
bliss, divine, 74
brahmacharya (studentship), 37
   in *raja yoga*, 98
Brahman, 13, 46, 63, 70, 78, 83,
   attainment of, 27
   Bliss as, 74
   consciousness as, 63-64
   defined, 13
   ideal of realization of, 67
   identity with *jiva*, 29, 30
   knowledge of 28, 73
   manifestations of, 74
   nature of, 61-62
   Ocean of, 53
   relationship to world of
      appearance, 28-29
   Sat-chid-ananda as, 65
   self or ego and, 39, 40
breathing:
   characteristics of, 107
   deep, 107-108
   processes of, 113
   rhythmic, 107-108
breathing exercises (*pranayama*)
   in *raja yoga*, 111
buddhi, 23

causation, aspects in *karma yoga*, 157-58

Chaitanya Sri, 135
chakras (spinal centres), 109-110-111
chastity (brahmacharya),
  raja yoga and, 98
chinmaya, 154
chit (intelligence), 87
chitta (mind-stuff), 23
  disturbances in, 95
  raja yoga and 93, 116-17
cleanliness *(soucha)*,
  raja yoga and, 100
concentration;
  means to realization through 60
  raja yoga and, 22-23
conduct, right, 183
Consciousness, 189
  divinity as, 61-62,
  evolution of, 189
  states of, 24-25
contemplative faculty, 36
  development of, 44-45
contentment *(santosha)*
  raja yoga and 97-100
  yoga and, 120
death, 76
deep sleep, 73
degeneration, danger of in spiritual life, 146-47
desire, need to control, 157
desirelessness, *jnana yoga* and, 91
desires, destructive, 183
detachment, 188
  attainment of, 49
devotion, one-pointed, 128
dharana (retention of consciousness), 95
  in *raja yoga*, 123
dhyana (meditation), 95, 123
  bhakti yoga and, 134
  raja yoga and, 123
dinata (modesty), 134, 143
disciple *(sishya)* instruction of, 56-57
discipline, in spiritual life, 182

disciplines, preliminary in *raja yoga*, 119-20
discrimination *(viveka)*, 38, 188
  importance of 48-49
  karma yoga and, 170, 171
dispassion;
  importance of, 49
  teaching of, 45
divine call, 47
divine life, attainment of, 184
divine love, 131-4
divinity, 2, 3, 5, 6, 7
  obstacles to 7, 9, 11

East and West, compared, 183-5
ecstasy:
  defined, 84
  jnana yoga and, 85
ego:
  concept of, 26
  function of, 25-26
  mind and, 189-90
  purification of, 189
emotion, proper direction of, 144-5,
emotions:
  bhakti yoga and, 126-8
  development of, 146
Existence, absolute, 70

faith *(sraddha)*, described, 51-2
fasting, 113
forebearance *(titiksha)*
  described, 51
freedom:
  karma yoga and, 158
  jnana yoga and, 84-5
  spiritual, 88

Gandhi, as *karma yogin*, 170
garhasthya (householder's life), 37
Gaudapada, philosophy of, 16-19
gifts, non-receiving of, 34, 99-100
God, 75
  conceptions of, 3, 179
  karma and, 156
  worship of, 187
Gopi maidens, 164

gunas, 161, 129
  characteristics of, 33
  described, 21
  meaning for man, 182
  spiritual development and, 181
  spiritual practices and, 115-6
guru:
  necessity for, 53, 128
  raja yoga and, 121
  relationship with, 56-7
  signs of a, 54
  types of, 54

Hindus, as lovers of God, 136-139
hope,
  non-entertainment of, 34
humanity, three types of, 172
hatha yoga 106
Ideal, struggle for, 52
ignorance, 45-47
  removal of, through purifying process, 63
inaction, as a discipline, 35
India, as spiritual centre, 183
inner discipline, need for, 101
Ishtam (Chosen Ideal) 143, 178, 190,
  bhakti yoga and, 127-8
  bhavasamadhi and, 151
  remembrance of, 134
  repetition of name of, 128
Iswara-pranidhana (surrender to God) in *raja yoga*, 103
Iswarakoti, 54, 88, 90
japam, 133, 143
jivakotis, 54, 89
jivanmukta (ever-free soul), 89 90
jnana yoga, 21
  fundamentals of, 70, 71
  goal of 26, 37
  summarized, 186

kalaha (quarrelling)
  bhakti yoga and, 141
Kapila, philosophy of, 22, 23, 24

Sankhya school and, 20-22
Vedanta and, 20-22
karana sarira, 23
karma, 129
  basic types of, 160-61
  classifications of, 159
  commentary on
    by Ramakrishna, 54
  compensatory, 158
  derivation of, 157
  environment and, 175
  good and bad, 159
  involuntary, 159
  law of causation and, 161
  samadhi after, 90
  sex and heredity and, 175
  simile of archer and, 161-2
karma yoga
  applications and, 168
  bhakti yoga and, 181-82
  defined, 156
  concentration and, 169
  freedom in, 160
  goal of, 156
  obstructions to, 180
  occupation and, 168
  proper work and, 175-76
  reincarnation and, 175
  requisites of, 171-72
  samadhi and, 180-181
  secret of, 157-58
  service to God and, 163-64
  stages of advancement in, 180
  subjective attitude in, 163-64
  success in, 179-80
  summarized, 189
karma yogin:
  characteristics of advanced, 181
  karmi (worker) and, 162-163
  man of action as, 170
kirtana (singing) in *bhakti yoga*, 141
knowledge, 72-73
  divine-71-72
  means of verifying, 6-7
  sources of, 3
kosas (sheaths), described, 23-24
Krishna, 136-39

authenticity of, 139
Ideal as, 136-37
Kriyamana karma, 161
kundalini, description of, 109-110
kundalini sakti, 105, 109
liberation (mumukshutwam), desire
    for 52-53
light, spiritual, 83-84
love, 126-27
    importance of, 140
    power of, 144
    search for Self as, 150

lust:
    bondage of, 138-39
    greed and, 183
madhura bhava, 151-52
mana (pique), in bhakti yoga 141
manomaya kosa, 24
manana (discriminative reasoning)
    in jnana yoga, 56, 58, 60, 66
mantram, 97, 128
maya, 14, 19, 20, 41
    defined, 14
    power of, 26, 30
medha (intellectual brilliance), in
    raja yoga, 98
meditation, 187
    beginning of, 50
    best times for, 116
    four steps of, 124-25
    places for practice of, 119
    raja yoga and, 123-24
    types of, 123
    way to Truth, 63
milana
    bhakti yoga and, 142
    defect of, 147-48
mind
    detachment of, 187-88
    nature of 24, 25, 122
    training of,
mind-stuff (chitta),calmness of, 95
Mira Bai, 120-21
monism, schools of, 15

Nag Mahasaya, 135
Narada, 132-33

negativism, 67
nididhyasana, jnana yoga and 56,
    59, 61, 66
nirvikalpa samadhi, 64, 88, 89,
    90, 123
nishtha (steadiness), in bhakti
    yoga, 133
niyama, 133
    bhakti yoga and, 133
    disciplines of, 95, 96
non-injury (ahimsa), in raja yoga,
    96
non-Self, false identification with,
    41, 42
non-stealing (ahimsa),in raja yoga,
    98
obstacles, elimination of,
    in karma yoga, 178, 179
obstructions, conquering of, 52
occupation, proper, 114
Ocean of Consciousness, 80
Oneness,
    Ocean of Brahman and, 75

paramahamsa, 153
Patanjali, 93, 95, 105
perfection
    attainment of, 189-90
    bhakti yoga and, 126
    desire and, 158
personality, harmony of, 188
philosophy, definition of correct
    181-82
philosophy of life, India and, 157
physical self, maintenance of, 9
posture (asana)
    benefits of, 104-105
    for meditation, 104-105
    raja yoga and, 104-106
prakriti, 22
pramana, 7, 15
prana, 107
    control of 107-108
Pranamaya kosa 24
pranas, 23
prarabdha karma, 152,161
pratyahara, 95
    raja yoga and, 123

prayer, 187
prema bhakti, 148-151
  characteristics, of, 149-50
  psychic powers, ignoring of, 120
puja (worship),
  bhakti yoga and 134
Purusha, 22
purva raga, 141
raganuga bhakti, 139-41
raja yoga,
  disciplines of, 187
  eight steps in, 95
  primary concern of, 98
  perfection in, 95
  summarized, 186

Ramakrishna, Sri 54, 88, 89,
    151, 152, 189-90,
reality, *jnana yoga* and, 82
reincarnation, 76,
  in Hindu psychology, 175
religion
  commandments of, 94-95
renunciation (*vairagya*), 49, 50, 51
  defined, 44

sad-chid-ananda 65, 78
sadhana (disciplines), in *bhakti*
    yoga, 130
Saint Paul, quoted, 71
sakhya bhava, 151
samadhi, in *raja yoga*, 124, 125
samskaras (tendencies), 175
samyama, 124
sanchita karma, 161
Sankaracharya, 17, 19
  four-fold disciplines of, 37-38
  nature of *Brahman* and, 61
  philosophy of, 18, 19
  qualifications for study of. 20
sannyasa (monkhood), 37
santa bhava, 151
santosha (contentment),
    raja yoga and, 100
sadguru, 54
  types of, 54
satyam (truthfulness),
    in *raja yoga*, 97

savikalpa samadhi, 123
Self, the, 79
  concept of, 4
  meditation on, 124
  Witness of body's activities. 41-42
self-abnegation, 131
Self-consciousness,
    freedom from 85-88
self-control, 49-50
self-surrender, 103, 104
self-withdrawal (*uparati*),
    as a discipline, 50
sense objects, defect of, 49
seva (service), 135, 143
sex consciousness, 98
sex instinct, 145
sheaths (*kosas*), 23-4
sishya (disciple), signs of a, 55-56
sukshma sarira, 23
siddhanta vakyam (spiritual state-
    ment), 86-87,
sincerity, in *karma yoga*, 170-171
smaranam (remembrance), 134,
    143
soucha (cleanliness),
    raja yoga and, 100
soul (or self), nature of 70
speech, control of, 33-34, 102
spiritual aspirants
  classified, 12
  disciplines described, 33-34
spiritual (psychic) centres, 110-112
spiritual practices
  favourable times for, 114
sraddha (faith) 142
sravana (hearing)
    bhakti yoga and, 141
sthula sarira, 22-23
surrender to God,
    in *raja yoga*, 103-104
swadharma, 175

tanmatras, 22
tapah (austerity) in *raja yoga*,
    101
tata bhava, 151
titiksha, (forbearance)
    described, 50-51

Turiyananda, Swami, 26, 50
tushti (satisfaction),
    danger of 147, 148
unity
    as ideal of philosophy, 67
    in variety, 68-70
universe,
    as divine manifestation, 31
upaguru, 54
upasana, in *bhakti yoga*, 133

Vaikuntha (heaven),
    bhakti yoga and, 154
vanaprastha (retirement), 37
vasana 10
vatsalya bhava, 151
Vedas, 126
vijnanamaya kosa, 24
viraha (longing),
    in *bhakti yoga*, 142
vishwa-premi (lover of the universe), in *bhakti yoga*, 150
viveka (discrimination), 37

Vivekananda, Swami, 147
    as author, 192-93
nirvikalpa samadhi and, 91
vrittis (thought waves),
    in *raja yoga*, 93

West and East, compared, 183-85
Witness
    realization of Self as, 41, 46, 47

    supreme, 41
work
    five aspects of, 176
    ideal of, 181
    perfection and, 158
    practice of unselfishness and, 187
    service to Self, 170
world, illusion of, 31
yoga, disciplines of, 101-102
yoga
    art of, 94
    consciousness and, 62
    defined, 12
    mysticism and, 197
    preparatory measures for, 113
    prerequisites for, 115-116, 119-120

Yoga Aphorisms of Patanjali 93
Yoga-Vasishta, 192
Yogas
    authorities on, 192
    combination of, 187
    definition by Vivekananda, 187
    harmony of, 186
    practices of 193
    scriptural references to, 192-193
    summarized, 186
    types of, 12